"With colorful examples of people experiencing an: identify with, David A. Clark expertly describes the cesses that underlie chronic anxiety. Even better, he __ dence-based strategies for counteracting each of these processes. A must-have book for anyone starting their journey toward an anxiety-free life."

—**Peter J. Norton, PhD**, professor of psychology at the Cairnmillar Institute in Australia, and author of *Group Cognitive-Behavioral Therapy for Anxiety* and coauthor of *The Anti-Anxiety Program*

"In *This Is What Anxiety Looks Like*, Clark writes an exceptionally clear and engaging volume on the personal stories of people suffering with anxiety. Working from the inside-out, Clark focuses on the key psychological mechanisms maintaining each person's specific anxiety cycle, and then carefully and elegantly demonstrates how step-by-step cognitive behavioral therapy (CBT) treatment strategies are delivered to target these mechanisms and reduce anxiety. This wonderful book is recommended for anyone seeking to better understand the nature, causes, and successful treatment of anxiety."

—**Neil A. Rector, PhD**, professor in the departments of psychiatry and psychological clinical science at the University of Toronto; director of the Forest Hill Centre for Cognitive Behavioural Therapy in Toronto, ON, Canada; and coauthor of *The Aging Well Workbook for Anxiety and Depression*

"This is what a self-help book looks like: modern, easy, and accessible to everyone. Written in an engaging and straightforward way without any jargon, it's packed with the latest insights on anxiety treatment. Perfect for the general population since it tackles the everyday anxiety we all face. Practical tips make it incredibly useful, and it's absolutely not tedious. It truly raises the standard for quality in self-help books!"

—**Claudio Sica, PhD**, professor of clinical psychology at the University of Florence in Italy, and author/editor of about ninety international publications on anxiety and personality disorders

"A brilliant decision to identify twelve core processes common in most anxiety presentations. The strategies identified to address these maintaining factors are sensible, easily understood, and spot-on! Clark's clinical wisdom and expertise are on full display. If anxiety interferes with how you want to live your life, you will find many helpful gems in these pages. Anxiety is manageable, and Clark shows the reader how to do it."

—**Maureen L. Whittal, PhD**, associate clinical professor at the University of British Columbia, and cofounder of Anxiety Canada

"In *This Is What Anxiety Looks Like*, Clark masterfully distills cutting-edge therapeutic techniques into easy-to-understand language. Real individuals (composites of Clark's cases) model different problems and their solutions, offering compelling demonstrations of how readers can address their own anxiety. Drawing on a lifetime of expertise, Clark weaves relatable stories, offering practical paths for self-help. There has never been a book like this before, so rich and yet so accessible."

—**Gary P. Brown, PhD**, professor of clinical psychology at the Royal
Holloway University of London

"This evidence-based book dissects anxiety piece by piece, offering relatable insights into its driving forces. Each chapter focuses on a specific anxiety-fueling element, explaining its mechanics and providing relevant case studies. The author's vast experience in writing self-help books is evident in the interventions offered, and provides accessible ways for readers to dismantle their anxiety. An invaluable resource for anyone seeking to understand and overcome their anxiety."

—**Guy Doron, PhD**, associate professor at Reichman University, director
of the ROCD research unit, and cofounder and chief scientist of GGtude

"Anxiety is a normal emotion, yet it is painful for those who suffer from its ravages. Renowned clinical psychologist David A. Clark has written an excellent step-by-step guide to help readers understand how a cascade of dysfunctional thoughts and behaviors can lead to a heightened sense of danger and worsen anxiety in the long run. His clear, incisive book—replete with clinical wisdom, rich examples, and practical tips—is a must-read for anyone who has struggled to overcome anxiety."

—**Lata K. McGinn, PhD**, professor of psychology in the Ferkauf Graduate
School of Psychology at Yeshiva University, cofounder of Cognitive &
Behavioral Consultants (CBC), and president of the World
Confederation of Cognitive and Behavioural Consultants (WCCBT)

"This is a wonderful and timely take on this topic for our times. David A. Clark has come up with an engaging and highly relatable way of communicating the things that matter most for solving and also learning to live with anxiety. A wonderful distillation of all his work over decades told in way that feels like a fireside chat—warm, wise, patient, and right on the science too. Even if you've read other books on the topic, there is so much that's fresh here."

—**Peter J. Bieling, PhD**, professor in the department of psychiatry and
behavioral neuroscience at McMaster University, and clinical consultant
for the Ontario Structured Psychotherapy Program

# This is what anxiety looks like.

**Relatable Stories, Targeted Solutions & CBT Skills for Lasting Relief**

David A. Clark, PhD

New Harbinger Publications, Inc.

## Publisher's Note

NEW HARBINGER PUBLICATIONS is a registered trademark of New Harbinger Publications, Inc.

New Harbinger Publications is an employee-owned company.

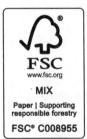

Copyright © 2024 by David A. Clark
New Harbinger Publications, Inc.
5720 Shattuck Avenue
Oakland, CA 94609
www.newharbinger.com

Cover design by Sara Christian

Acquired by Ryan Buresh

Edited by Amber Williams

Library of Congress Cataloging-in-Publication Data on file

Printed in the United States of America

26    25    24

10    9    8    7    6    5    4    3    2    1          First Printing

To the many individuals in my practice who shared with me their personal stories and experiences with anxiety and worry, I am truly grateful. You taught me much about the many faces of anxiety, and together we learned how to manage this difficult emotion. This book would not be possible without your insights, courage, and determination to grow beyond your personal turmoil.

# Contents

# What to Expect

Michelle felt on edge more days than not. Since childhood, anxiety had been a dominant emotion in her life. She had been a nervous child who avoided risks and preferred the safety and security of her family and a couple of close friends. Adulthood brought with it increased responsibilities of work and family, which caused a dramatic rise in her general state of tension, agitation, and apprehension. Now, Michelle can't stop thinking about potential problems and the possibility of negative consequences resulting from her actions and decisions. She feels overwhelmed much of the day and wonders if the demands of life are too much. She's impatient, easily frustrated, and irritable. Even the smallest obstacle can ruin her day, making it impossible to think through issues in a calm, rational manner. Overwhelming anxiety has killed any chance of joy, with moments of happiness being few and far between.

Gina's experience with anxiety is very different. For starters, she was more confident and resourceful than Michelle was, taking life's difficulties as problems to be solved. Gina knew what she wanted from life. She had meaningful work, a loving family, and close friends. As an intelligent, determined, and well-organized person, Gina had a strong sense of control over her emotional well-being and purpose in life. But all this came to a crashing end one Saturday afternoon while she was shopping in a crowded supermarket. Gina usually gave herself lots of time to do a *big family grocery order, but on this day she was running late to pick up her nine-year-old daughter from ballet class. She chose the shortest cashier line only to find the customer ahead exceptionally slow and confused. Suddenly, she felt a wave of intense heat wash over her body, followed by dizziness, shortness of breath, chest pain, and unsteadiness. It felt like she might faint. Fortunately, there was a chair close by, and Gina sat there for several minutes until the dizziness passed. She left the grocery store with a splitting headache and was considerably late picking up her daughter. It was an embarrassing ordeal because Gina's daughter was upset, and Gina had to pay a late-pickup fine to the ballet instructor. Worse, since that incident, Gina has been gripped by a fear of having another panic attack. She's baffled by the panic attacks and is worried she'll have another for no apparent reason. Her belief in her emotional stability has been shattered, and she now avoids crowds and other public places for fear of having another spell. For the first time in her life Gina is dealing with anxiety and a fear of losing control of her emotions.*

*Dwayne is a loner who feels uncomfortable around others, especially his own age group. Even back in elementary school Dwayne was quiet, shy, and had only one close friend. He was not into sports or other school activities. He developed an intense interest in gaming, spending long hours in his room playing on his devices. Now a successful game developer, Dwayne still feels uncomfortable in social gatherings. When entering a group setting, he immediately feels conspicuous, like everyone is looking at him and thinking, Here comes the nerd, a real loser. He feels tense, awkward, and self-conscious. When he tries to speak, his mouth feels dry, his tongue thickens, and his voice becomes high-pitched and squeaky. Most often he's at a loss for words, which he takes as evidence of social incompetence. This whole experience is so distressing for Dwayne that he avoids interaction with others as much as possible. He's able to work from home, so his only in-person contact is with immediate family. But lately Dwayne feels nervous even in these family gatherings. His world is shrinking, leaving him in a perpetual state of loneliness and despair.*

We all know what it's like to feel anxious. Even if you can't identify with Michelle, Gina, or Dwayne, it's likely you've had other experiences of anxiety. There are many circumstances in everyday living that can make us feel nervous or anxious. Maybe it's traveling on your own, preparing for a job interview, meeting an important person for the first time, taking an exam, confronting someone about a wrong, or feeling trapped in a crowd. All these situations can cause us to feel tense and nervous. Because anxiety is such a common emotion, it's easy to assume we know what it is. But do you really know the "nuts and bolts" of anxiety—what's behind the nervous, agitated feeling that makes it so persistent and distressing?

Experience and knowledge are not the same. You can experience the feeling of anxiousness but not understand the underlying processes that drive the emotion. *This Is What Anxiety Looks Like* delves into the basics of anxiety, offering treatment strategies that target the processes responsible for the emotion. Let's begin by agreeing on what we mean by anxiety. It is the anticipation of threat or danger to ourself or people we care about. Anxiety has two undeniable characteristics: it's a distressing emotion, and it involves the totality of our being, affecting the way we think, feel, and act. It can involve a physical threat, like a fear of cancer, or it could be a psychological threat, like a person's fear of being embarrassed or shamed. So let's take a moment to unravel this complex experience we call anxiety.

## This Is Anxiety

The following is a diagram for understanding the thoughts, feelings, physical sensations, and actions that characterize anxiety.

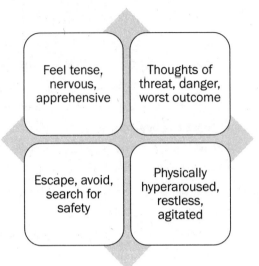

Feel tense, nervous, apprehensive

Thoughts of threat, danger, worst outcome

Escape, avoid, search for safety

Physically hyperaroused, restless, agitated

Figure 1

Often, we're most aware of how anxiety makes us feel. Let's say your day is going quite well. It was an easy drive to work, you had a nice chat with coworkers at the beginning of the day, and you were able to get some work done. Then you get an email from your manager reminding you of a presentation you're scheduled to make to senior management at three this afternoon. You'd forgotten about the presentation and you're not prepared. Instantly your mood changes. You suddenly feel tense, stressed, nervous, fearful, and maybe frustrated and irritated. It feels like you're in panic mode. We've all been there, and it's not at all pleasant. In fact, the feeling of anxiousness can be so distressing that we'll do practically anything to get relief from this keyed-up state.

In times like these, it becomes apparent that anxiety also changes the way we think. When anxious, we become preoccupied with threats to our physical or psychological well-being. You can think of nothing else but the threat or danger you imagine could happen to you or your loved ones. A young mother drops off her eighteen-month-old child at daycare for the first time. She's been dreading this day for a while and now finds she can't concentrate at work. Her mind is filled with thoughts about her baby. *Is she crying hysterically for mommy? Are the daycare workers taking good care of her? Am I a bad mother for sending my child to daycare?*

With a mind flooded with worrisome thoughts about "bad things" that could happen, this young mother feels more and more anxious until she decides to text the daycare, inquiring about her child's well-being.

When we're anxious, we tend to exaggerate the likelihood and severity that something bad could happen. Michelle, for instance, tended to see insurmountable problems and difficulties at every turn in her life. Gina found her worries about panic attacks became especially acute in public places when she was most conscious of herself. Dwayne often imagined embarrassing himself in front of others. Although the threat was different in each case, the tendency to assume that misfortune is very likely and that the consequences would be severe is a way of thinking that drives up anxiety.

Another characteristic of anxious thinking is the belief that we're incapable of dealing with the problem or threat that's causing our anxiety. A high-school student was convinced she could never be a good student because she was unable to deal with her intense test anxiety. An executive in his sixties felt anxious about retirement because he didn't think he could handle the financial insecurity and unstructured day. And many young adults feel anxious and then avoid dating because they're convinced they can't deal with intimacy or possible rejection. All sorts of human experiences entail some level of risk and stress—but that stress will feel much worse if anxiety has you believing you're helpless and unable to deal with life's difficulties.

To illustrate how thinking affects feelings, consider dental anxiety. Most people can recall at least one unpleasant, even painful, trip to the dentist. But only a few people develop an intense fear and avoidance of dentists. Most of us feel some anxiety, but it doesn't stop us from going. So what's the difference? The .person who develops an intense anxiety about dentist appointments thinks: *The pain is too much to bear, once in the dentist's chair I'm trapped and can't leave, I hate the oral anesthetic injections, I can't breathe with all the instruments in my mouth.* And so they decide to wait until the toothache becomes unbearable.

However, this is not how the vast majority of people think about dental appointments. Their anxiety is much less because they think: *I can take the pain because it's only momentary, good oral hygiene is important to me. Once I get the injection of lidocaine, all the rest is relatively pain free, and if I get anxious or feel like I need to catch my breath, I can ask the dentist to pause for a couple of minutes.* Notice how each way of thinking either drives up anxiety or drives it down.

Finally, there's the matter of how we act when we're anxious. Have you heard of the fight-or-flight response? This is how we all react when feeling afraid. We either stand and confront the danger or we run, escape, or avoid, trying to put as much distance as possible between us and the source of our fear. The fight-or-flight response is automatic; it can overtake us before we know it. And often, when it comes to anxiety, flight responses—escape and avoidance—are the most common. When we perceive a threat and feel anxious, escaping or avoiding that threat becomes the quickest and most effective way to find relief—at least in the moment. But there's a problem. The more we avoid whatever it is that makes us anxious, the longer the anxiety persists. Escape or outright avoidance means we never learn that the threat is not as bad as we think, that we can tolerate the anxiety, and that we can deal effectively with the situation.

For example, some people with health anxiety refuse to see their doctor for fear a symptom might indicate a serious illness. In this case avoiding doctors and hospitals perpetuates health anxiety because you never find out if a symptom is serious or benign—and you never confront the anxiety you feel in such a way that you learn you actually can get through it, even if it feels like you can't. If you're afraid of having an anxiety attack in crowds, then avoiding crowds seems like the logical solution. But avoidance has a way of spreading so over time you avoid more and more places because you're thinking they may be too crowded (like restaurants, grocery stores, retail stores). Again, you don't give yourself the chance to learn that you can actually deal with the anxiety you feel, no matter how intense it may be.

That said, escape and avoidance are not the only actions that can make anxiety worse. Taking substances, like alcohol or drugs, makes anxiety worse by artificially lowering agitation without your having learned skills to actually tolerate the emotion. Reassurance seeking, the practice of seeking reassurance in a bid to assuage your anxieties when they arise, may provide some temporary relief, but that relief is short-lived, and often the anxiety returns as strong as ever. Your bid for reassurance can also strain your relationships. Rumination, which is a tendency to overanalyze the causes of anxiety, rarely provides new insights and only makes the anxiety more intense. As you can tell, there are many ways we react to anxiety that are ineffective at best and at worst actually strengthen the intensity and duration of anxious feelings.

## How Anxiety Affects the Body

We are all well acquainted with the physical aspect of fear and anxiety. It's the complete opposite of calm and relaxed. Your body becomes hyperaroused because of sudden activation of your autonomic nervous system. You know the telltale signs: increased heart rate, tightness in your chest, shortness of breath or breathlessness, general muscle tension, but also a feeling of being weak or unsteady, lightheadedness, dizziness, maybe blurred vision, feeling of nausea or upset stomach, and the like. You might experience different combinations of these physical symptoms when you're anxious, and some will be more intense and frightening than others. But whatever the physical symptoms of your anxiety response, they'll all have two properties in common: they mobilize the body for fight or flight in response to a perceived danger, and they are very uncomfortable. In fact, it's physiological hyperarousal that makes anxiety feel so distressing, and for many it is the physical symptoms of anxiety they find most intolerable. This, incidentally, is why so many people turn to chemical relief from drugs or alcohol when feeling anxious. They're seeking some way to calm their body, to neutralize what feels like a complete loss of control.

You might think that the physiological arousal we see in anxiety is fairly straightforward. But nothing could be further from the truth. Take roller coasters. Some people love them, others are terrified. I recently had a roller coaster experience with my six-year-old granddaughter. She loves them, but I have more fear and anxiety. Reluctantly I agreed to go with her and the rest of the family after seeing the excited anticipation in her eyes. Here's the interesting thing. My granddaughter and I had the same physical experience but an entirely different emotion. We both experienced heart palpitations, tense muscles, rapid and shallow breathing, dizziness, some nausea, and diluted pupils ("eyes like saucers"). However, we had very different interpretations of the physical symptoms. She loved the physical arousal, taking it as a sign of excitement, fun, and joy. For her it was a wonderful "adrenaline rush." For me, those same sensations were a sign of anxiety, an uncomfortable feeling that only subsided when I could see the end of the ride.

What this story reveals is that when it comes to anxiety reduction, the presence of physical symptoms is much less important than how you interpret them. Do you view them as tolerable and acceptable, or are they so frightening that you try to eliminate them as quickly as possible? As you can see, there's more to anxiety than a feeling. Getting to know the basics of anxiety and how to tailor interventions to deal with these underlying processes is the key to effective treatment.

## Cognitive Behavior Therapy for Anxiety

Cognitive behavior therapy (or CBT) is an action-based talk therapy that focuses on the most pressing problems you face in everyday living. CBT is a structured, goal-directed psychological treatment that spends less time on your past, and more on the present-day contributors to emotional problems like anxiety. It's based on the assertion that *the way we think or understand a situation and how we respond to it determine how we feel*. If you change how you think about yourself and the problems you face, and you change how you cope with them, then your emotional reaction changes as well. Cognitive behavior therapists have developed many interventions that focus on changing the thoughts, beliefs, and behaviors that cause anxiety. You'll learn about these strategies in the following chapters. The CBT view of anxiety is seen in this illustration.

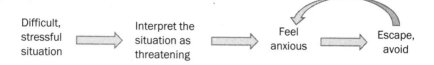

Figure 2

Consider a difficult situation all too familiar to most of us: waiting for a job interview. There are two ways to deal with this situation. One person feels such intense anxiety that they decide to cancel the interview despite really wanting the job. The second person also feels anxious but attends the interview and is offered the job. Why is anxiety so devastating for the first person but not the second? The answer lies in how they interpret the impending job interview. The first person thinks, *I'm going to blow this interview, my mind will go blank and I'll make a fool of myself, the anxiety will be so bad that everyone will see I'm a wreck, there's no way they'll hire me.*

Can you see how thinking this way about the interview would escalate the anxiety and cause the person to cancel? In this instance, escape and avoidance has a two-way effect. When we're anxious we want to escape the difficult situation, but escape and avoidance also makes anxiety worse in the future.

The second person thinks, *Okay, I know I'm anxious, but most people are anxious about job interviews. In the past I've been anxious and still functioned. The interviewers will be understanding and expect me to be anxious, besides I've prepared for this interview and my competence will show through my anxiety. I suppose the worst that can happen is not getting the job.* Can you see how the second person's way of thinking is much healthier than the first persons? CBT uses well-researched and proven strategies to help people change their thinking and way of coping, so they better tolerate anxiety and reach important life goals and values.

# What You'll Get from This Book

If you're curious about CBT and whether it can help with your anxiety, then this book is for you. It's written for people with different types of anxiety and worry who are wondering if CBT strategies can help them manage their emotional distress more effectively. It assumes you're new to CBT and so offers a crisp, concise introduction to anxiety and its treatment. It is not a workbook with complicated exercises and worksheets, nor does it provide lengthy, detailed explanations about psychological processes and concepts. Instead, it introduces you to the most powerful tools of CBT through the lives of individuals just like you who struggled with anxiety and worry. (These individuals are all composites of real people I've treated with CBT for anxiety; identifying characteristics have been changed to protect their privacy and confidentiality. Also the interventions they used are reconstructed and intended for educational purposes only.)

In the book you'll find twelve short, story-based chapters, each of which highlights a basic feature of anxiety or worry and provides three to four unique CBT interventions that are known to be effective agents of change for that specific feature of anxiety. You'll learn about the CBT approach by reading about the anxiety and worry of others and how specific intervention strategies eased these difficult experiences. By learning how others used CBT to overcome their anxiety, you'll be able to use these strategies on your anxiety and worry. Because each chapter centers around a detailed life story that illustrates a specific process in anxiety, I think you'll find this book more engaging and relatable than conventional therapy self-help books.

You may find some chapters more relevant than others, and that's okay. Spend more time reading the relevant chapters and practicing their interventions. I've provided some free downloadable worksheets at http://www .newharbinger.com/53165. You'll find these useful when practicing the interventions described in the following chapters. You can do a light read of the less relevant chapters without sacrificing the flow and organization of the book.

Learning about anxiety starts with the next chapter on the toxic effects of anxious anticipation. Have you noticed how easily you get worked up even thinking about having to do something that makes you anxious? You are anticipating some troubling situation and you can feel the anxiety rise before it even happens. This is one of the earliest processes that drive up anxiety, so it makes sense to consider interventions that target anticipation.

# CHAPTER 1

# Too Much Thinking

Anticipatory anxiety: *a feeling of apprehension,
worry, or dread when thinking about a future
experience, situation, or circumstance that is
expected to cause significant fear, anxiety, or panic.*

Remember the last time you dreaded going somewhere or having to do something you really didn't want to do? Do you recall how anxious you felt even thinking about this looming obligation? It might have been giving a presentation, meeting an important person for the first time, having a job interview, going to a party full of strangers, or traveling alone to a foreign country. If you have a specific fear, just thinking about doing something related to that fear can be distressing. If you're afraid of flying, for instance, you could be anxious and worried for weeks before taking a necessary flight. And if you have health anxiety, you might feel very anxious and upset waiting for medical test results.

The anxiety we experience before confronting a fearful or distressing situation is called *anticipatory anxiety*. It's an important part of the anxiety cycle, as illustrated below:

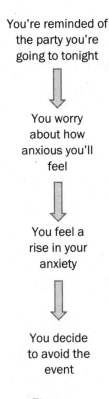

You're reminded of
the party you're
going to tonight

You worry
about how
anxious you'll
feel

You feel a
rise in your
anxiety

You decide
to avoid the
event

Figure 3

If you worry about how anxious you'll feel at a future event, like a party where you'll have to meet people—and you think you need to impress them—you'll experience a rise in anxiety as you worry about the event. The anxiety can become so intense it drives you to back out of the obligation altogether. Because of this process, anticipatory anxiety is responsible for causing much of the limitation and reduced quality of life we see in anxiety. Many of the people I've treated tell me their anxiety during anticipation was much greater than the anxiety they had during the dreaded event. That is, **thinking about doing it was much more distressing than actually doing it.** This was Jessica's experience. Her anticipatory anxiety was so great that she felt defeated before she even got started.

## Jessica's Story

Anxiety became a significant problem for Jessica as she approached her first year of college. Leaving home for the first time is traumatic for many seventeen- and eighteen-year-olds but it was especially difficult for Jessica because she was shy and introverted by nature.

Her anxiety about leaving home started the moment she received an acceptance letter from a prestigious fine arts college in a distant city. Although several months away, she experienced an acute anxiety attack as she read the letter to her parents. Her heart raced, her hands shook, her mouth went dry, she felt dizzy and lightheaded, and she felt breathless as if not able to get enough air. She had to sit down to finish the letter, and her voice became so faint her parents could barely hear. At one point Jessica felt detached from the moment, with the strange feeling that somehow this moment was not real. But of course she knew this was no dream. She was actually reading an acceptance letter. She had been admitted to the college of her dreams and with a scholarship that made her acceptance of the offer all but inevitable. Everyone would think "she was out of her mind" if she turned down this once-in-a-lifetime opportunity. And yet what flashed through Jessica's mind at that moment was *Be careful what you wish for*, followed by *I can't possibly do this. It's way too terrifying.*

Jessica had five months to experience intense anticipatory anxiety about starting college. Hardly an hour passed that she didn't think about it and what it would be like. With each passing day, the anxiety built as the departure date loomed closer and closer. Whenever Jessica thought about college, she imagined nothing but catastrophe. She was convinced she'd have intense anxiety day after day being forced to live and interact with students she didn't know. She was certain she'd be unbearably homesick within the first week. She would be forced to attend orientation week, which, with all the scheduled social activities with unfamiliar people, felt like it'd be her absolute nightmare. She also worried she'd become known as the weirdo who spent all her time alone and other kids would talk about her behind her back. All in all, Jessica's tendency to think only of threat, failure, and misery when she imagined the first weeks of college made her anticipatory anxiety much worse.

Jessica had always thought of herself as emotionally fragile. She had difficulty tolerating anxiety and was easily frightened, so she tried to avoid anything that was novel or unpredictable. Rationally, she knew that millions of young people leave home for college and they learn to adjust and even thrive. Still, she was convinced she was just different. Not only would she experience unrelenting anxiety, and probably embarrass herself both in class and residence, but she thought anxiety and sleeplessness would leave her tired, so much so that she'd be run down and probably susceptible to colds, COVID-19, and influenza. She kept thinking to herself, *How can I possibly get through all this? It's just too much.*

Ultimately, Jessica found herself debating whether to go away for college at all. Perhaps she'd be better off staying home and attending a local junior college. From a career perspective, the choice was obvious: go to the school she'd been accepted into. But Jessica was able to invent a variety of reasons for staying home, even as she knew she'd probably regret that decision the rest of her life. And in the end, the back-and-forth debate did nothing but increase her anticipatory anxiety. She then tried what felt like a more proactive strategy, to make plans on how she'd cope with the first month away from home. She even brainstormed with her parents. But the suggestions were never very convincing, because at the end of the day Jessica knew she was about to experience one of the most distressing periods of her life. It felt like no amount of troubleshooting could assuage the anxiety for long.

Does Jessica's experience sound familiar to you? Possibly there have been big changes in your life that led you to periods of intense anticipatory anxiety, like deciding to start a new job, beginning a new relationship, having a baby, deciding to retire, or moving to a new community. Or maybe anticipatory anxiety is an everyday occurrence for you, associated with the more routine activities of daily living—being in crowds or in public places, driving unfamiliar routes, attending appointments, trying to resolve conflicts with family members or friends, being home alone, and so on. But anticipatory anxiety is just that, anticipation (an expectation), whether the issue is big or small. It'll be driven by the way of thinking that drove Jessica's anxiety. You can use strategies that help people like Jessica with their anticipatory anxiety. Strategies like discovering a more realistic way to think about the anticipated situation, practicing effective coping skills when anticipatory anxiety strikes, and learning to take a more accepting, tolerant approach to anxiety.

# Hit the Brakes on Harmful Anticipation

## 1. Practice Realistic Thinking

Jessica realized that the anticipatory anxiety she felt in the months before leaving for college was all in her head. She knew that the way she imagined the first weeks of college was making her feel anxious months before the actual experience. But when she tried to figure out exactly what was driving her anxiety, her mind seemed to race from one anxious possibility to the next. To get a handle on her high anticipatory anxiety, Jessica could start by identifying precisely what frightened her most about leaving home and starting college. After considering all the challenges associated with being a first-year university student, Jessica realized her anticipatory anxiety centered on two core fears: *I don't know how to make friends* and *What if the anxiety becomes unbearable?* So any work she did on anticipatory anxiety had to focus on these two core issues.

Next, Jessica felt she needed to be specific about the worst-case scenarios she thought about, during periods of anticipatory anxiety. What exactly was it she was afraid of, and why? She thought it helpful to write out the specific details of her nightmare scenarios. For her fear of making friends, she wrote:

> *Everyone will ignore me. If I walk in a room, the other girls will glance at me and then continue talking to each other. I'll have to sit alone with no one to talk to. I'll feel so uncomfortable. If I try to break into a conversation, I'll say something stupid. My voice will be faint and shaky. Everyone will know I'm anxious and think, What's wrong with her? It'll be so embarrassing. Eventually I'll slink back to my room feeling totally defeated, ashamed of myself. I'll end up having one of my uncontrollable crying spells. But even there I have no privacy because of my roommates. I'll have to take a long walk and find some isolated spot on campus to cry my heart out.*

Jessica's nightmare scenario about feeling anxious went like this:

> *I'll be anxious every waking moment. No matter what I do about my anxiety, nothing helps. My anxiety will be greatest when I'm around other students, but I'll also feel anxious in class because I don't know anyone. There is a lot of group work in arts courses, which I find very troubling. I can't imagine any situation that would relieve me of feeling anxious, except maybe walking alone off campus. The anxiety will be punctuated with terrible panic attacks that scare me a lot. I won't be able to sleep because of worry about the next day. I'll be so anxious and exhausted most days that I'll be pushed to the brink of a nervous breakdown. My mental health can't take the strain and I'll have to quit before the end of the first month.*

After writing out the worst-case scenarios, the next step had two parts. Jessica started by writing down the best possible outcome she could imagine about starting college. She wrote:

*I arrive at university, and much to my surprise, it turns out to be an amazing experience. Everyone is so kind and accepting. The other first-year students go out of their way to include me. I'm invited to more social events than I could ever imagine, and my roommate is a quiet, studious person just like me. It feels like we've been lifelong friends. After the first week of some apprehension, I feel completely at home with little anxiety to no anxiety most days. I never realized life could be so awesome.*

Jessica quickly realized the best possible outcome was pure fantasy, but it was more difficult for her to believe that the worst possible outcomes she'd imagined before were just as unlikely. But in reality, as Jessica will likely discover when she's actually at college—and as you'll likely discover too—the situations we find ourselves in are more likely to be somewhere in the middle of the two extremes of absolute worst or best outcome.

From there, Jessica's next step was to think deeply about a more realistic outcome that fell somewhere between the worst and most desired outcomes. Here's what she wrote down.

*The first couple of weeks will be quite difficult. Everything will feel strange and I will likely struggle to initiate a conversation with fellow students. My anxiety will be high most days and I may have a couple of panic attacks. No doubt I'll have more bad than good days as I'm settling in. But the anxiety will fluctuate, and it'll probably be less intense as time goes on. There are hundreds of first-year students and many of them will be quiet and shy like me. Maybe I can meet one or two of them in class or at a resident event. We can band together. I don't have to be friends with the loud, confident party girls. I can be me and learn to be comfortable with who I am.*

The final step in this intervention was to list the reasons or evidence why the worst-case scenario is unlikely to happen and then list the reasons or evidence why the more realistic outcome is likely to happen. Each time Jessica feels anticipatory anxiety build, she could work on this final step so she is more focused on the realistic outcome rather than the worst-case scenario. Dwelling on an unlikely "catastrophic" outcome will make her feel more anxious about leaving for college. Now she can consciously redirect her attention out of those patterns of rumination to the more likely outcome, and along with the next strategies, quell her anticipatory anxiety.

## 2. Maximize Your Coping Potential

While the first CBT strategy is a good start, thinking about the most realistic college experience will not be enough to stem Jessica's high anticipatory anxiety. She must also create a coping plan for dealing with her moderate to high anxiety. You can think of the coping plan as a way to put into practice the realistic outcomes you imagined in the last exercise.

Jessica's coping plan must focus on the two core aspects of her anticipatory anxiety that she identified earlier: how can she manage the high levels of anxiety she'll experience at college, and how she can deal with her social inhibitions. Her coping plan needs to include a few steps:

a.  Learning to mindfully observe her anxious thoughts without judgment or effort to suppress the thoughts, both of which contribute to high anxiety.

b.  Learning to counter catastrophic thinking with more realistic predictions about what might happen.

c.  Focusing on controlled breathing, to counter the physical symptoms of anxiety.

d.  Utilizing meditation and other calming skills when she senses her anxiety rising.

For her anxiety about meeting new students and connecting with her peers, Jessica could do some social skills trainings that include:

a.  Practicing how to initiate and maintain a casual conversation with peers.

b.  Exploring ways to improve her social media footprint.

c.  Learning to be more assertive.

d.  Practicing techniques to improve her verbal and nonverbal communication skills.

When Jessica had high anticipatory anxiety, she was focused on how anxious she'd feel the first few weeks of college. Instead, shifting her focus from anxiety to coping will lessen her anticipatory anxiety. But just reminding herself of her coping plan will not be enough. She had five months before college to practice the skills in her coping plan. Practice coping with anxiety during the anticipatory phase will strengthen her anxiety management skills and boost her self-confidence to face those first weeks of college.

## 3. Go with the Flow

Anxiety is an emotion, and like all emotions, it's a way of feeling that can change from one moment to the next. Often, trying to control an emotion, especially one like anxiety, can make it worse rather than better. Instead, riding the wave of anxiety—allowing your feelings to rise and fall on their own—is much better than trying to swim against the current. Jessica can use this strategy, of surfing the waves of her feelings, whenever her anxiety rises as she's thinking about leaving for college. Instead of wrestling with the anxiety and trying to eliminate it, she can accept that she's feeling anxious and let it fade naturally, on its own. She might even do some self-talk like:

> I notice I'm starting to feel anxious again about college. It's perfectly natural to have anxious thoughts when imagining what September will be like. Who wouldn't have some anxiety about something so important and unknown? I know my mind gets carried away with exaggerated thoughts of intolerable anxiety, loneliness, and embarrassment. It's impossible to fight against these thoughts because they are in my imagination; I'm not in college yet. Instead, I'm going to sit on the sidelines and just watch these thoughts float through my mind like clouds in the sky. I'll sit here and watch the thoughts for ten to twenty minutes

*until I feel like I've done enough watching. Then I'm going to get up and continue on with my day because I can only have an impact on the present. My imaginary college experience is thinking about a future that will end up being different from what I'm imagining at the moment.*

You'll see Jessica is validating her own feelings (*It's perfectly natural, Anyone would be anxious about a change this big, I know my mind gets carried away,* etc.). She's not afraid of her feelings or trying to eliminate them. She's also recognizing what she will do, rather than fearing what she imagines she can't do (*I'm going to sit on the sidelines and just watch these thoughts float through my mind*). And she places a limit on the amount of time she spends anxiously thinking about the future, resolving to get up and do something else after a predetermined time period. In this way, Jessica is limiting the effects of anxiety and learning to live in the present, even when feeling anxious about the future.

## What You Can Do

Anticipatory anxiety is the earliest phase of the anxiety cycle. It can take you down a path toward intense anxiety where you may decide it's better to avoid than face your fear. You imagine unbearable anxiety, decide to avoid it, but this can feed into a vicious cycle of more frequent and intense anxiety experiences, not to mention a reduction in your daily functioning and life satisfaction. That's why it's important to "nip it in the bud." By practicing strategies that slow down anticipatory anxiety, you'll be working on one of the earliest contributors to problematic anxiety.

The three interventions in this chapter are designed to help you disengage from your anticipatory anxiety. The realistic thinking strategy targets the root cause of anticipatory anxiety: imagining the worst and being convinced your only option is to avoid. (See http://www.newharbinger.com/53165 for the worksheet.) As you'll discover, rarely does the worst (or the best) ever happen. Instead, it's somewhere between these two extremes. And most people believe they can tolerate some risk, but if you're always imagining extreme risk or threat, the future will seem overpowering. Your anticipatory anxiety will ease up if you're convinced a more balanced, realistic alternative is most likely to happen.

What's more, when we become overly focused on our emotions, anticipatory anxiety is worse. *I can't stand the anxiety,* we might think. *I've got to get a grip on myself. This is going to push me over the edge.* The second and third interventions in this chapter are designed to shift your perspective from this emotion-focused approach to a problem-focused perspective. Instead, you may think, *What can I do right now to prepare for what I think will be a difficult situation in the future?* And you might think, *I can start to build up my anxiety tolerance today rather than wait for what I dread in the future.*

If you tend to feel anxious when you think about the future, you can practice adopting an anxiety-acceptance mindset today. Leaving home for college at eighteen years of age is a momentous life event, but Jessica can learn to put the brakes on anticipatory anxiety by changing how she thinks about her future, refocusing on the present, and reinterpreting any queasy feeling about the future as a natural, acceptable response to an impending life challenge. You can use the same strategies she did to address your anticipatory anxiety head-on too.

CHAPTER 2

# Anxious About
# Being Anxious

High anxiety sensitivity: *a heightened intolerance,
even fear, of feeling anxious because of the belief that
anxiety symptoms have significant adverse physical,
social, or psychological consequences.*

**Can you be anxious about being anxious?** If you've ever Googled phobias, you know that we can develop a fear of almost anything. But what about a fear of anxiety? Can we have a fear of an emotion? The answer is yes, and it's called *anxiety sensitivity*.

Anxiety sensitivity consists of three core elements: hypersensitivity to signs of anxiety, inability to tolerate the physical symptoms of anxiety, and a belief that anxiety is harmful.

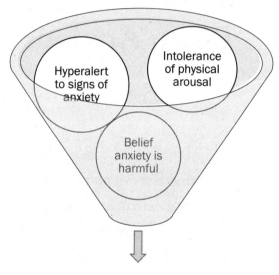

**High Anxiety Sensitivity**

Figure 4

It is often the physical symptoms of anxiety that people with high anxiety sensitivity fear most. Anxiety sensitive people will sometimes avoid exercise, even when physical arousal is to be expected, because they don't like being out of breath, sweating, or feeling their heart race. And of course, physical arousal that occurs out of the blue, for no apparent reason, is especially frightening. Given this heightened sensitivity and fear of physical arousal, the anxiety sensitive person is on the lookout for any signs of anxiety. We call this hypervigilance for any feeling, symptom, or circumstance that might portend anxiety. Once they detect even the possibility of anxiety, the anxiety sensitive person will take evasive action. This is because of the third element of anxiety sensitivity: a belief that anxiety is harmful to one's health.

Do you see yourself in this description? Are you overly sensitive to the symptoms of anxiety? Could this make your anxiety experiences more intense than a less sensitive person? Possibly you know you overreact to anxiety, but you don't know how to change. As you will see in Shandra's story, high anxiety sensitivity made her emotionally volatile and unable to deal with many of life's challenges.

## Shandra's Story

By her forty-seventh birthday, Shandra had ticked all the boxes. She had a loving family, an affectionate and understanding husband, good health, lots of friends, and financial security. After graduating from university, she eventually got a job with a large financial firm and worked her way into senior management. Shandra had the "right stuff" to be successful. She was smart, industrious, ambitious, and personable.

But Shandra was an intense person. Her day was filled with stress because of the pressure she put on herself to achieve. Her drivenness was combined with a tendency to experience strong emotion. Some might say she was rather high-strung. More often than not, Shandra experienced the extreme ends of emotion. In happy times, Shandra was exuberant; if sad or blue, she was really down in the dumps. She could easily be brought to tears over the smallest ordeal. So when Shandra felt anxious or fearful, it is not surprising it was experienced with great intensity.

Shortly after her birthday, Shandra started having severe migraines. She generally took her health seriously, being very cautious about her diet and getting regular exercise. The migraines caused her considerable anxiety. They didn't respond to anything she tried to use to treat them, and they interfered in her ability to work and enjoy life. She started to feel anxious about her health, and then it happened. One day while taking her morning walk, Shandra experienced a panic attack. Suddenly, she felt waves of hot flashes, like electricity, course through her body at the same time that a profound weakness caused her to lose balance. She felt lightheaded and dizzy, as if she might faint. She stumbled to the nearest bench and sat down. She didn't know what was happening. Was she having some type of spell related to her headaches? Could it be an aneurysm or some type of mini-seizure? She was alone and a couple of miles from home. She started to cry uncontrollably, thinking she might be dying. It seemed like an eternity, but probably only fifteen minutes or so had passed when Shandra realized she needed to call 911. The paramedics arrived quickly and decided she needed to be taken to the hospital. After several hours of testing and consultation, it was determined that Shandra had had a panic attack.

That incident occurred nine months ago and since then Shandra has been afraid of having another attack. She's come to believe that anxiety can unexpectedly escalate into a severe emotional state, even panic. So she pays very close attention to her emotions and physical state. When she wakes in the morning, she thinks, *Will anxiety ruin my day? I hope I don't feel anxious.* As soon as she opens her eyes, she begins to take stock of her feelings. Certain sensations like feeling tense, restless, tired, or emotional cause Shandra to worry that anxiety will soon follow. Any sudden and unexpected physical symptom, like chest discomfort, lightheadedness, or nausea, magnifies her fear exponentially. In fact, she's become so concerned about feeling anxious that she can think of practically nothing else during the day. Her sleep has deteriorated, dominated by worries of never gaining control over the anxiety.

What was most intolerable, to Shandra's mind, was her loss of emotional control. Her emotions had always been intense, but she'd learned to manage them. Now, though, when anxiety took hold, she found she would shake and cry uncontrollably. This often occurred around family, friends, even coworkers, so Shandra often felt embarrassed by what observers might label as "her antics." She often complained to others about "the dreaded anxiety." At first, people offered her sympathy and reassurance. But soon, they lost patience with Shandra's emotional outbursts. She was now having more anxious days than not, and once it started it lasted most of the day. Frequently during therapy sessions Shandra had crying episodes, wringing her hands, and saying her life was ruined by anxiety.

Shandra's panic attack was a watershed moment. She had always been an enthusiastic, energetic, highly productive person who could deal with stress and uncertainties to reach her objectives. But all that changed with the panic attack. Her self-confidence and resourcefulness were replaced with self-doubt, emotionality, and fear.

In the sections that follow, you'll discover the strategies that Shandra—and you—can use to overcome the fear of anxiety. These include learning that anxiety is an ever-changing emotion that can be faced as a momentary state, reducing excessive focus on emotions, becoming more comfortable with physical arousal through strenuous exercise, and being more accurate at labeling your negative emotional states.

# Conquer Fear of Anxiety

## 1. Rethink Anxiety

Anxiety is a normal emotion. It's no more possible to live anxiety-free than it is to live without sadness, frustration, or anger. But Shandra had come to view anxiety as a dangerous emotion, a feeling that she had to avoid or eliminate because it was such a destructive force. To overcome this fear of feeling anxious, Shandra started by changing her understanding of anxiety. Ultimately, her goal is to accept that anxiety is a normal emotion, one that's not dangerous and can even be helpful depending on the circumstances.

Her work to reorient her thinking about anxiety begins with a simple self-monitoring exercise, to gain a more accurate understanding of her anxiety. Shandra keeps track of her daily anxiety by giving herself an anxiety score each hour of the day. First, she makes a note of what she was doing in that hour and her level of productivity (ability to accomplish). Then she rates her anxiety level during that hour using a 0–10 scale, where 0 = "no anxiety," 5 = "moderate anxiety," and 10 = "intense anxiety." Her record might look something like this:

| Hour | Activity | Anxiety Rating |
|------|----------|----------------|
| 7:00 a.m. | Rushed, getting ready for work (a little productive) | 2 |
| 8:00 a.m. | In traffic, driving to work (a little productive) | 4 |
| 9:00 a.m. | At work, doing emails (enjoyable and productive) | 1 |
| 10:00 a.m. | Planning meeting with team (frustrated but productive in the end) | 7 |

It's important that Shandra keep this exercise very brief, maybe taking only one minute per hour to complete it. (See http://www.newharbinger.com /53165 for the worksheet.) After two or three weeks, Shandra can review the data she collected to look for several trends as indicated by the following questions.

a. Was she surprised to find more experiences of low to moderate anxiety than high anxiety?

b. When anxiety was low to moderate, was she more productive or did she experience more enjoyment than she might have expected?

c. Were the experiences of high anxiety more or less devastating than she expected? Were they always devastating, or was some of the high anxiety less negative than expected?

d. Did high anxiety always last longer, or were there times when low anxiety was more enduring?

e. Regardless of its level, was the anxiety she experienced ever helpful in dealing with a difficult situation or solving a problem at work or home?

By doing this self-monitoring exercise and delving more deeply into the data she collected, Shandra will learn that anxiety is a normal emotion that varies in strength and ebbs and flows throughout the day. She will learn that anxiety isn't just a devastating emotion that must be feared. Rather, she can live with and adapt to anxiety just as she does to the other positive and negative emotions in her life.

## 2. Counter Self-Fulfilling Prophecy

Shandra's fear of anxiety had become a self-fulfilling prophecy. She started each day predicting that at some point she'd feel intolerable, distressing anxiety and then reacted poorly to the slightest indication she was "feeling off," which ensured a rise in her anxiety level. How could Shandra counter this self-defeating spiral into intolerable anxiety? The goal is to change the prediction from *I'll experience intolerable anxiety that will ruin my day* to *I'll experience some varying levels of anxiety throughout the day—and I'll cope with them just as I cope with other changes in my emotions.*

One strategy to achieve this change is to observe how others deal with their anxiety. Excessive self-focus is a major contributor to anxiety, so it can be therapeutic to turn your attention outward and observe others. Shandra practices being an astute observer of her coworkers, friends, or family when they were performing a task (making a presentation, initiating a conversation, introducing themselves). She considers questions like: Do they appear anxious? Does anxiety impact their performance or have other negative consequences? Do people judge them negatively for being anxious? How do they manage or accept their anxiety? If she learns to observe others in this way, rather than focusing on herself, Shandra might be surprised to learn that anxiety is common in other people, they acclimate to it, and it seems to have no lasting effect. This brings her to the obvious revelation: *If others can treat anxiety as a normal, unwanted negative emotion, so can I.*

What's more, once Shandra begins to start the day by making a prediction that she'll experience some anxiety of varying levels, this changes her perspective on her own anxiety from the thought, *I hope I don't get anxious,* to the more grounded and realistic, *I know I'll experience some anxiety, so I need to focus on living my life effectively even when anxious.* She can practice using various strategies that help her work productively, connect with family and friends, and meet the many demands of daily living while still feeling anxious.

The following are some strategies that can improve Shandra's tolerance of feeling anxious—and yours.

a. **Maintain task-oriented focus.** When you're anxious about being anxious, there's a tendency to become overly focused on your feelings at the first sign of anxiety. To counter this excessive self-focus, Shandra needs to learn to notice when she's falling into this cycle and then consciously shift her attention back to whatever she's actually doing. Each time her mind drifts back to thoughts like *I feel so terrible,* she will acknowledge her feelings and then gently turn her attention back to the task at hand, rather than letting the feelings pull her further along the path of anxiety and worry.

b. **Practice calming, patient, methodical coping.** It's well known that taking a few deep breaths, slowing down, and taking a situation one step at a time can counter the impulsivity and hyperarousal of anxiety. Shandra can learn meditative breathing and remind herself to slow down, breathe, and focus on the next step in dealing with a difficult situation or problem.

c. **Never avoid, quit, or make excuses because of your anxiety.** A person with high anxiety sensitivity will be tempted to make an excuse to themselves or others to justify escaping or avoiding the prospect of feeling anxious. Even though it was out of character for her, Shandra found herself doing this time and again after her panic attack. She now excused herself from certain work responsibilities, turned down invitations to parties or other social activities, and stopped going to the gym for fear her anxiety would spike. But now, rather than avoid potentially anxiety-provoking situations entirely, Shandra decides to try to navigate the situation with her anxiety, rather than letting the anxiety or her fear of its consequences call the shots. She knows that only by challenging automatic thoughts, like *I can't stand feeling anxious, nothing is worse than feeling anxious,* can she learn greater tolerance and acceptance of this negative emotional state.

## 3. Physical Exercise

No doubt you're very familiar with the health benefits associated with regular exercise, but did you also know that aerobic exercise can reduce anxiety? If you think about it for a moment, this makes perfect sense. As we learned at the start of this chapter, if you're anxious about being anxious, you won't like the physiological arousal you experience when anxious. But aerobic exercise—activities like walking, running, cycling, or swimming—which involves working out your cardiovascular system, will dramatically increase physiological arousal (increased heart rate, rapid breathing, tense muscles). When you engage in twenty to thirty minutes of aerobic exercise, you are forcing yourself to experience the same physiological sensations that you so dislike when anxious.

Shandra had been a walker before her first panic attack. Combined with a careful diet, this had been enough to keep her healthy. But now that Shandra had become fearful of anxiety, she had developed an aversion to becoming physiologically aroused—and so she'd stopped walking. Now it was critical that she resume exercise as part of her treatment for high anxiety sensitivity—and develop a more intense aerobic exercise program to really experience the symptoms that so disturbed her when she was anxious.

This involved a few steps. First, Shandra spoke with her family doctor to rule out any medical condition that would preclude increased physical exercise. She then decided to meet with a physical trainer to determine her level of fitness and design an individualized aerobic exercise program that would meet her needs. She also realized it would likely take many weeks of consistently working her program before she'd experience any anxiety-reducing benefits. As her trainer advised her, she'd have to face three obstacles that can erode motivation:

a. **Believing that exercise is optional.** Rather, Shandra would need to consider exercise essential for her physical and mental health.

b. **Too little time for exercise.** Shandra would need to make time for exercise in her busy schedule and stubbornly guard that time.

c. **Letting discomfort drive her to fall off her routine.** Expect that the pain and physical discomfort of exercise will be more intense for her due to anxiety sensitivity but remind herself that she's strengthening her cardiovascular system through training and not putting it at risk.

## 4. Emotion Reattribution

Anytime Shandra felt upset, frustrated, or became tearful, she automatically assumed anxiety was just around the corner. She was quick to label any emotional distress as anxiety. Because of her fear of being anxious, this tendency to attribute any upset to anxiety made matters worse. It caused her to become inwardly focused and overly concerned with avoiding any further emotional escalation for fear of an anxiety attack. In reality, Shandra often mislabeled the emotion she was feeling as anxiety when it was more likely stress. We call this a *misattribution error*.

To correct this misattribution error, Shandra can write down what's happening during times when she's feeling distressed, as a way to really observe her experience for its truth rather than jumping to conclusions about it. For example, say one day she suddenly bursts into tears. She can ask herself, *What's happening at this moment? Am I dealing with a problem and not making progress? Am I feeling overwhelmed, rushed, out of control?* If the answer to these questions is "yes," she'll know she's likely experiencing stress. Alternatively, she can ask herself, *Am I worried about something in the future?*

*Am I thinking I'll be unable to deal with this future problem? Am I stuck in "what if" thinking? Am I trying to solve future problems that don't yet exist?* If the answer to any of these questions is "yes," then she may be experiencing anxiety. Through this intervention, Shandra learns that she often mislabels stress as anxiety. And once she learns this—*Oh yes, I'm feeling stressed*—she can then focus on dealing with the stressful situation rather than focusing on not getting anxious.

## What You Can Do

Like Shandra, is fear of feeling anxious driving up your experience of anxiety? If so, this is *anxiety sensitivity,* and it's probably causing you to have more unwanted experiences of anxiety. Let's say you're frightened of dogs. It's not hard to believe that you might have more negative dog experiences than someone not frightened of dogs. The same goes for fear of anxiety. You might have more anxiety experiences that are intolerable than a person with low anxiety sensitivity because your fear increases your awareness of feeling anxious. That's why it's important to raise your level of anxiety tolerance and eliminate your fear of feeling anxious. This will have a positive effect of reducing the frequency and intensity of your anxiety episodes.

Practicing the skills you learned about in this chapter (viewing anxiety as a fluctuating momentary state, doing less monitoring of your feelings, being more comfortable with physical arousal, and accurately labeling your negative emotions) will help. There are also a few more issues to consider when working on fear of anxiety.

a.  Be patient with yourself. The longer you've struggled with high anxiety sensitivity, the longer it'll take to reduce your fear. And confronting fear takes courage. It's one of our toughest challenges, whether it's a fear of something external, like animals or insects, or a feeling like anxiety.

b.  The first exercise suggests you monitor your anxiety level for a couple of weeks to learn about the natural flow of anxiety. It's important to stop self-monitoring after a couple of weeks. People with high anxiety sensitivity are hyperaware of any signs of anxiety, and you don't want to reinforce this problem with excessive self-monitoring.

c.   Maintaining motivation for cardiovascular exercise is tough for anyone. I've been running for almost twenty-five years, and it's still easy to "fall off the wagon." Doing regular aerobic exercise is even harder for people with high anxiety sensitivity. There are many self-help resources available on how to make physical exercise a daily routine. I encourage you to take advantage of whatever resources you need to boost your motivation because regular aerobic exercise can play a major role in reducing your fear of the physical symptoms of anxiety.

d.   Possibly you find one or more of the physical symptoms of anxiety the most distressing part of feeling anxious. Whether it's a racing heart, breathlessness, muscle tension, lightheadedness or the like, strengthening your tolerance of these symptoms will be important to reducing your "fear of anxiety." To help you in this endeavor, you'll find an extra chapter entitled *Anxiety That Feels Explosive* at http://www.newharbinger. com/53165 that provides a case example and exercises for dealing with the physiological hyperarousal of anxiety.

# CHAPTER 3

# The Great Escape

Avoidance: *to restrict activities of daily living to reduce the possibility of triggering intolerable feelings of fear, anxiety, or worry.*

Procrastination and avoidance are as natural as breathing. Early in life we learn to stay clear of anything that is distressing or makes us feel uncomfortable. We seek out situations that generate positive feelings and avoid situations that cause negative emotions like sadness, fear, frustration, or anxiety. If making a speech causes you intense anxiety, you'll avoid public presentations. If you're nervous or anxious about driving, you may limit how much you drive. And if you have test anxiety, you might choose less important courses that don't require tests.

Common sense tells us to avoid distressing experiences and their triggers. But what if anxiety is so frequent and so intense that you start avoiding things that are necessary for living? Why would someone avoid activities and responsibilities that are so important to living a full and satisfying life? Would not the cost of avoidance be so much greater than its reward? Of course, costs and benefits are very much in the eye of the beholder. I recall treating an older man with severe agoraphobia. He had not left his house for twenty years because of the fear and panic he would feel upon opening his front door and stepping outside. In his mind being housebound was less costly than facing his fear.

This chapter focuses on two responses to anxiety that psychologists consider together: escape and avoidance. *Escape* refers to leaving an anxiety-provoking situation before anxiety declines naturally, and *avoidance* is the refusal to approach a situation believed to be anxiety-provoking. Both responses are driven by the anticipation of terrible anxiety you won't be able to tolerate and a preference for relief and (perceived) safety:

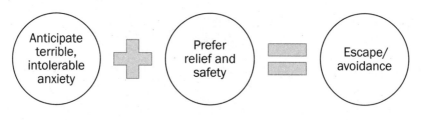

Figure 5

If you believe you're likely to feel intense anxiety in a crowded supermarket and you are fearful of feeling anxious (see chapter 2), you will prefer the safety and security of staying home. You'll depend on someone else to do your grocery shopping or you'll have groceries delivered to your door. If someone convinces you to go grocery shopping, you'll probably leave (escape) at the first sign of discomfort because you want to prevent anxiety escalating to an intolerable level. This two-pronged process leading to escape and avoidance dominated Jamal's life. He started avoiding just a few uncomfortable situations but gradually it grew to include more and more activities of daily living. Now he's incapacitated by anxiety and avoidance, and it's threatening to derail his hopes and dreams.

## Jamal's Story

Jamal could remember a time when he was easygoing and carefree. He had fond memories of high school where he was popular and well liked because of his athletic skills, friendliness, love of music, and easy time with most academic subjects. He had lots of friends, a secure and loving family, and a comfortable living standard. But all this changed when he left home for college. For the first time in his life Jamal felt insecure. Both the sports and the classes were much more demanding than he expected, and he didn't have the support of old friends.

It was during the first weeks away from home that Jamal experienced serious anxiety. He was a few minutes late for an introduction to calculus class. It was a huge class held in an auditorium that seated over 500 students. It was jam-packed, with only one seat available in the center of the classroom. The lecture had already started, and Jamal had to squeeze past a dozen students to get to his seat. It seemed like everyone was looking at him, and for a second the lecturer appeared to stop until Jamal found his seat. After a few minutes of trying to take notes on a very boring but complicated computation, Jamal felt an intense wave of heat wash over his body from head to foot. At the same time he felt dizzy and lightheaded, his heart rate accelerated, and he felt like he couldn't breathe. Once before, he had had the same feelings during an intense practice on a very hot day; he'd almost passed out. Later, he'd attributed the experience to dehydration. But now he was just sitting in class, so why the same out-of-control feelings? Was he about to pass out now? If he did, it would disrupt the class, and it'd be incredibly embarrassing. He had to leave. So, he got up, and despite the stares this earned him, he quickly ran out of the class. Once he escaped the building and got his first gulp of fresh air, the physical sensations started to subside. It took Jamal fifteen minutes to get back to his room. By the time he got there, the symptoms had passed, and he felt a strong sense of relief. But Jamal knew he had missed an important class.

After that, Jamal became increasingly anxious in crowds, social gatherings, and public places. He stopped attending large classes and tried to keep up with online tutorials and lectures. The dining halls made him feel extremely self-conscious because it seemed like everyone noticed he was eating alone, so he relied more and more on bringing take-out meals to his room. He avoided dorm social events and also stopped responding to the invites of the couple of guys he'd gotten to know during orientation week. Jamal even stopped posting to his social media because he had become a loner, and he didn't want his old friends to know he was struggling. Being alone in his room felt like the only safe place. The ordinary tasks of college life seemed daunting. Also, Jamal was afraid he'd have another anxiety attack, so an escape into safety seemed like the best option. In this way, avoidance became his preferred way of coping with what felt like terrible possibilities.

Does Jamal's experience sound familiar? Avoidance can take many forms. You might avoid any situation where you fear your anxiety will draw the attention of others. Or you might avoid situations, like crowded stores or elevators, where you feel trapped. You might try to avoid certain feelings like embarrassment or guilt, and some people try to avoid disturbing thoughts like thinking about sex or betrayal. Others seek to avoid unexplained physical sensations like a racing heart. Despite the variety of triggers, what is common to all is a desire to escape feeling anxious or avoid the possibility of anxious symptoms. Has your life been shrinking because of a fear of feeling anxious? Have isolation and avoidance become your "great escapes"? If so, take a look at three interventions that Jamal can use to achieve victory over escape and avoidance, and reclaim his life. These are a systematic program of exposure to triggers of avoidance, strategies to strengthen resilience to anxiety, and coping skills for getting through the increased anxiety experienced during exposure.

# Strategies to Conquer Avoidance

## 1. Confront the Fear

By a certain point in Jamal's first year, the way his life had been diminished by anxiety and fear started to really bother him. It was a trip home after his first semester that really spurred him to change. His younger brother had asked him if college was cool; he lied and said yes—and the lie gnawed at him, leading him to realize something had to change. He decided he had to confront his fear, at least to some extent, rather than let it drive him.

He went to his university counseling center to a see a therapist, who advised him to begin by assessing which situations caused him anxiety and how much. Some situations caused Jamal severe anxiety, so he always avoided them. But there were other situations he would sometimes avoid and at other times was able to face, albeit with considerable effort. He also noticed that he was more likely to avoid when tired or stressed, and less likely when accompanied by a friend or family member who made him feel safe—or to whom he felt an obligation to keep going, even when anxiety reared its head.

When avoidance is variable as it was for Jamal, it's important to get a better understanding of your escape and avoidance responses as a first step toward confronting your fear and anxiety. Creating a trigger list is an easy, straightforward way to do this. In creating his trigger list, Jamal wrote down every situation, event, person, activity, or experience that would be difficult to engage with because of anxiety. Most people with anxiety are able to create a list of twenty to thirty situations or experiences. These situations are likely to generate varying levels of discomfort and avoidance, so the next step was for Jamal to rate each situation on a 0–10 scale, where 0 meant "would not avoid," 5 meant "likely to avoid about half the time," and 10 meant "likely to always avoid," and then to arrange the situations in descending order, with the situations he was most likely to avoid on top and the situations he was least likely to avoid at the end. Here are some examples from Jamal's avoidance hierarchy, along with his ratings.

| | |
|---|---|
| Late for class, finding a seat in the middle of a front row. | 10 |
| Going to a football game and sitting where my dormmates can see me. | 9 |
| Start attending class in-person. | 7 |
| Eating alone in crowded dining hall. | 6 |
| Going to dorm social event. | 5 |
| Speaking to another student before class starts. | 4 |
| Starting a text thread with an old friend back home. | 2 |

The next step is called exposure therapy, and it involves facing your anxiety and discomfort in a planned, orderly manner. It takes considerable courage and determination to do this type of therapy because it involves deliberately making yourself uncomfortable. But exposure is the most powerful psychological treatment for fear, anxiety, and avoidance. As Jamal's therapist told him, when he expressed apprehension about it, if Jamal was willing to put the time into this strategy, he'd see big changes in his anxiety and avoidance.

To get the most from exposure, Jamal needed to plan out each exposure exercise before he did it. He knew he needed to start with a situation he avoided that was moderately anxiety-provoking. So, he decided to work on going to the dining hall for lunch and supper. This was a good starting point because avoiding the dining hall was proving to be expensive and the takeaway meals were unhealthy. On his therapist's advice, he broke the exposure down into several steps. He started by going to the dining hall at off-hours because it was less crowded and his anxiety would be lower. He did this twice a day, every day for two weeks. As his therapist predicted, Jamal's anxiety dropped to almost zero by week two. He then gradually changed the time, so he eventually ate in the dining hall during peak hours. At first his anxiety was very high, but he was determined to tolerate the discomfort. Eventually he became more comfortable with the dining hall and decided it was time to tackle another avoided situation in his hierarchy. He chose to work on attending large lectures like Introduction to Calculus. He started by ensuring he got to class ten minutes early so he could sit in the back row. He did this for a couple of weeks until he felt less anxious. Next, he decided to sit at the end of a row halfway up the lecture hall, and so on until he was able to sit anywhere in the crowded classroom.

## 2. Increase Anxiety Tolerance

To break the avoidance habit, you'll also need to tolerate greater amounts of anxiety and discomfort. This will be true whether or not you intentionally ramp up your anxiety through exposure therapy. It's almost impossible to reduce avoidance if you're still overly sensitive to feeling anxious. Greater anxiety tolerance will allow you to let your anxiety decline naturally as you confront all the anxiety triggers you've been avoiding. For Jamal his therapist explained that he'd need to *embrace* his anxiety while doing his exposure exercises for them to be effective.

Two strategies are key to increasing anxiety tolerance. The first is *mindful acceptance of anxious thoughts*. Jamal was told to pay close attention to the anxious thoughts that intruded into his mind when he confronted his anxiety triggers. He could record the main anxious thoughts on the notes app of his phone. He then asked himself several questions about these thoughts:

- Am I making a catastrophic prediction (like *I'm going to faint/collapse/start screaming/etc.)*?

- What's the worst that's most likely to happen when I'm feeling anxious?

- Do I have more control over my emotions than I think?

- I can tolerate pain, so what makes me think I can't tolerate some anxiety?

After asking himself these probing questions in anxious moments, Jamal practiced accepting the thoughts that arose when he was anxious, rather than struggling against them. He let them sit in his mind, even if it felt a little stressful to let them be there, and waited to see the outcome if he did nothing. Most of the time, nothing terrible happened and he got through the anxiety situation much better than he expected.

The second strategy is *mindful acceptance of physical symptoms*. When he was feeling anxious, Jamal worked to take the perspective of a detached observer on any physical symptoms of anxiety he experienced. For example, he often noticed his heart rate increased and he sweated more when he was anxious. But now, instead of assuming these symptoms were abnormal and a sign he was out of control, he thought of all the other times his heart rate accelerated and he sweated. Working out at the gym, running up a flight of stairs, or rushing to class all caused the same physical symptoms and yet they didn't scare him. And of course, rationally, Jamal knew he was a young man in good health so there was no reason why a higher heart rate or sweating was dangerous. So, Jamal resolved to simply observe the symptoms as if he was watching them occur in another person. He thought to himself, *Well, I guess my heart wants to beat faster and my sweat glands are working overtime. That's okay, I'll just let my body do its own thing.*

## 3. Manage Anxious Feelings

Jamal had at his disposal a few more strategies to help manage his anxiety. Generally, strengthening anxiety management skills helps you build confidence that you can handle situations that may seem overwhelming. And when you feel confident in your emotion-regulation skills, your fear, anxiety, and avoidance often decline.

The first anxiety management technique is called *grounding,* and it involves focusing attention on the details of your physical environment. It's a form of distraction that also functions as a reminder that the present moment is safer than the anxious mind thinks. *Diaphragmatic breathing* is another technique that people often use to counter the tendency to hyperventilate when feeling anxious. (See *Anxiety That Feels Explosive* at http://www.newharbinger.com/53165 for more details.) Again, this involves breathing normally through the nose at a four-second rate of inhalation and exhalation. *Slowing down* is a third coping strategy for anxiety. When Jamal felt anxious around others, his speech and physical activity accelerated because he wanted to get through the anxious experience as quickly as possible. But being quick and impulsive can make you feel more anxious and out of control. So, Jamal practiced saying to himself, *Take it slow, slow down, pay attention to what you're doing,* to counter his tendency to rush.

## What You Can Do

After taking a hard look at your anxiety and worry, are you like Jamal? Does escape and avoidance contribute to your problem with anxiety? Has your life become smaller because of all the situations and experiences you now avoid? No doubt you've noticed that once you started avoiding, you became less tolerant of anxious feelings and more concerned about safety and relief from anxiety.

If you've struggled with anxiety for years, escape and avoidance may be so automatic that you hardly give them a second thought. Your default response may be to avoid even if you merely anticipate an anxiety-provoking situation. You make excuses and convince yourself it's better to avoid a situation altogether than to get all stressed out. The avoidance habit will be hard to break, but it begins with being honest with yourself. It starts by realizing that avoidance is making your anxiety problem worse, and that failing to confront your anxieties is not good for your health or quality of life. Then, you'll want to come up with a trigger list, just as Jamal did, and work through each of the situations on your list in a series of exposures. (See the worksheet available at http://www.newharbinger.com/53165.)

You'll need to start your exposures with the situations on your list that are least anxiety-provoking and keep working at it until you feel less anxious and more confident in the situation. Then it's time to progress to a slightly more difficult situation. It's impossible to say how long this process will take, so be kind and patient with yourself. Also, don't be afraid to reach out for support from a therapist or other professional if you feel it'll be useful and you have the means. After all, confronting fear is one of the hardest things you can do.

Sometimes avoidance takes the form of *overcontrol,* an excessive effort to suppress unwanted thoughts and feelings. We all experience unwanted thoughts and feelings that suddenly pop into our awareness. It could be a negative feeling like guilt, shame, or remorse, or it could be a selfish, disgusting, or immoral thought. As you'll know from reading Jamal's story, and others in this book, we can't avoid thoughts and feelings in the same way we can avoid external situations—but we can become preoccupied with controlling these thoughts and feelings, trying to push them outside our awareness or eliminate them altogether. When we do this, we are engaging in avoidance. The best antidote for this type of *mental avoidance* is acceptance. That is, you learn to let go of control and allow your mind to wander wherever it chooses. As it wanders, even into territory you would prefer to avoid, you can acknowledge what is happening and then gently bring your attention back to a task at hand. Dialing back on excessive mental control is another way to overcome avoidance. And generally, you'll find that, when you let go of attempts to control your thoughts, they'll roll on through your mind of their own accord, where trying to make them go away, paradoxically, makes them more intensely objects of your attention.

If you've tried exposure therapy in the past, or if you've used some of the anxiety management strategies mentioned in this chapter but haven't achieved a desired benefit, again, consider working with a therapist. Most people find that the advice and support of a mental health professional makes all the difference in the world when they're working on avoidance.

And remember, the longer you've been avoiding, the more difficult it can be to reverse this debilitating coping strategy. Chronic avoiders may find they need more detailed, step-by-step instruction or a professional's support to break the escape/avoidance habit. But you can do it—and you'll find materials to support you in this effort in the resources at the end of this book.

# CHAPTER 4

# Down but Not Out

Anxious helplessness: *strongly held beliefs that you're emotionally fragile, weak, and incapable of tolerating thoughts, feelings, and experiences of unintended fear, anxiety, or worry.*

Does life feel overwhelming because you can't catch a break from anxiety or worry? Maybe your difficulty with anxiety has made you believe you're emotionally fragile, not as strong or resilient as others. As you look back over your life, has anxiety changed you into a person you never dreamed was possible? Perhaps you remember a time when you were more engaged with life—confident, independent, and resourceful—but anxiety has taken a terrible toll and now you're filled with fear, self-doubt, and inse-curity. When anxiety causes us to think we're weak and vulnerable, we call this *anxious helplessness*.

Anxious helplessness causes people to become avoidant and highly dependent on others to manage their heightened fear and anxiety. If you believe you're weak and emotionally fragile, you're more likely to avoid any-thing that makes you feel uncomfortable. As the avoidance spreads, you become more and more dependent on your partner, family members or close friends to look after your day-to-day needs. Ultimately, anxious helplessness can become a vicious cycle:

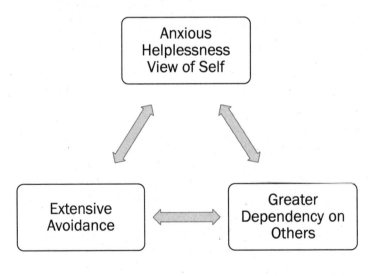

Figure 6

Anxiety causes you to think of yourself as weak and vulnerable; you then avoid situations and are more dependent on others because you're convinced you're weak and incapable of dealing with life; this in turn reinforces your belief in being weak and vulnerable. This vicious cycle defined Rafael's life, driving him to the point of utter despair.

## Rafael's Story

Rafael's life has been a struggle since his early twenties, but the last ten years have been especially heartbreaking. After graduating from university with a degree in electrical engineering, Rafael was hopeful for his future. He landed a great job with a large engineering firm, married Anna, and settled into the suburbs located near a large midwestern city. Anna was able to find her dream job as an elementary school teacher and within a few years the couple had two children. Despite all this good fortune, a dark shadow lingered in the background. Starting in his teen years, Rafael struggled with anxiety and worry. He coped with the help of medication and occasional therapy but at times it felt like he was barely keeping his head above water.

As the pressures of work, finances, parenting, and the myriad other responsibilities of daily living continued to mount, Rafael could feel his anxiety build. He was beginning to experience more anxious days than not. His sleep had deteriorated and he was falling into long periods of intense worry. He'd also started experiencing the physical symptoms of anxiety like heart palpitations, shortness of breath, dizzy spells, and headaches. This caused him to worry about his health. Rafael struggled with weight and high blood pressure, which were causes of concern considering his family history of cardiovascular disease. Then one day Rafael had the most intense panic attack he'd had in years. What happened next proved to be life-changing.

The panic attack happened at work. After medical investigations ruled out any cardiac abnormality, Rafael took some time off work and tried to recuperate at home. Unfortunately, the incident left Rafael feeling anxious most of the time and, despite an increase in his medication, unable to get a good night's sleep, making the anxiety even harder to deal with. He lost any confidence in himself altogether and became overwhelmingly fearful of another panic attack.

For Rafael, feeling as exhausted and unwell as he did now, the presence of anxiety became proof that he was emotionally fragile, that he was not as strong as others, and so he needed to take extra precautions to protect his health. He became incredibly aware of the things he felt triggered his anxiety and decided he needed to cut these activities out of his life to reduce the stress. It started with cutting out social activities. It then progressed to avoiding all public places because of his concern that he might feel anxious. After three years of unrelenting anxiety and avoidance, Rafael ended up practically housebound. Fortunately, he remained employed by convincing his employer to let him work from home even before the COVID-19 pandemic.

Rafael's condition had a profound effect on Anna. He became highly dependent on her to take care of most of the family responsibilities. This meant she did all the grocery shopping, driving, transporting the children to their activities, as well as all chores and responsibilities outside the home. And it meant she could no longer travel or take vacations, go out to restaurants, meet with friends, or attend synagogue activities because Rafael felt anxious when alone at night. Even in the rare times she was able to get him to commit, he was likely to pull out at the last minute. Anna found she was always making excuses for Rafael, saying he was not well enough to attend functions.. As the months passed, the dependency took a toll on the couple's marriage. Rafael knew he was placing a terrible burden on Anna but what could he do? He needed her, but Anna was beginning to buckle under the strain. The arguments and conflict increased, and there was now talk of a trial separation.

Does Rafael's story sound familiar? Are avoidance and dependency a big part of your experience with anxiety? There are many reasons for Rafael's problem with anxiety. One of the most significant was his belief that he was weak, vulnerable, and emotionally fragile. Because Rafael had come to see himself in this way, he believed he had to avoid getting anxious or stressed, and he needed to depend on others to care for him. This belief in personal helplessness caused Rafael to remain trapped in anxiety and fear. But fortunately, anxious helplessness is a false set of beliefs. It's a distortion of who you really are, caused by persistent anxiety. Let's take a look at three strategies

Rafael could use to rediscover his strength and resilience and adopt a healthy view of himself: rediscovering past skills in dealing with moderate levels of anxiety, phasing out his dependency on Anna, who had become a safety signal for him, and creating opportunities to practice greater independence and assertiveness.

# Strategies to Rediscover Yourself

## 1. Revealing Your True Self

Because Rafael believed he was weaker and more emotionally vulnerable than others, he thought he had to minimize his stress as much as possible, which led him to depend on others for most of the tasks of daily living. But Rafael's view of himself had become distorted by his anxiety. To counter his anxious helplessness, he first needed a more realistic, balanced understanding of who he was: what we call our *self-concept*.

Rafael's work on his self-concept began with rediscovering who he really is. Is he as weak and helpless as he believes? The following rediscovery exercise was useful in this regard. He divided a blank page into two columns labeled "Past Experiences of Coping with Anxiety" and "Strategies and Skills I Used to Tolerate Past Anxiety." (See http://www.newharbinger.com/53165 for the worksheet.) In the first column, Rafael listed times in the past when he felt anxious but coped with or tolerated emotional distress. It's important to be as specific as possible. In the second column, he listed any strategies he used in the past to tolerate and "push through" his anxiety. Rafael wrote the following items in the first column:

**Past Experiences of Coping with Anxiety**

- Interviewing for my current job

- When I proposed to Anna

- Applying for our first mortgage

- The initial appointment I made with the doctor about my chest pain

- Driving in heavy traffic in Chicago

And here's what he wrote for the second column:

**Strategies/Skills Used to Tolerate Past Anxiety**

- Focused on preparing for the interview

- Believed she'd say "yes"; realized the time was right

- Went through with application process even though I felt nauseous

- Convinced myself I'd feel relieved once I got reassurance from my doctor that it wasn't a serious medical condition

- Gave myself extra time, listened to calming music, didn't do a lot of lane changing

In writing out these lists, Rafael realized he had many anxious experiences in the past and was able to get through them just fine. He was reminded of some coping strategies he used to ride out these anxious experiences. Clearly, he is not as weak and helpless in the face of anxiety as he's come to believe. In the past he relied on himself rather than others. When you're overcome by persistent anxiety, and avoidance and dependency become your primary modus operandi, it's easy to forget your past coping strategies—and just how capable you can be.

## 2. Phasing Out Dependency

As it stood, Rafael felt embarrassed by his excessive dependency on Anna and it was putting a strain on their marriage. He knew that weaning himself off this dependency would play a critical role in regaining his self-confidence and believing that he wasn't a helpless victim of anxiety. He also knew it could improve both their lives significantly if he could stick with it.

Ultimately, we learn best through experience. A gradual "extinction program," in which Rafael listed all the situations in which he relied on Anna and tackled them one by one, was the best way for him to reduce his dependency. So Rafael starts by listing all the anxiety-provoking situations in which he feels he needs Anna. (See the worksheet at http://www.newhar binger.com/53165.)

These might include driving, supermarkets, malls, restaurants, being alone in the house at night, meeting a friend for coffee, and the like. Next, he arranges these situations from ones he absolutely can't do without Anna to situations where he'd prefer to have Anna close by but he might be able to go through them on his own, albeit with some discomfort.

In the next step, Rafael selects the situation at the bottom of his list and, for one or two weeks, engages in this activity daily or at least several times a week, testing his ability to do them without Anna nearby. For example, he could choose "staying home alone at night for at least one hour." Anna often takes the kids to their evening activities, and Rafael usually comes along to avoid being at home alone. Instead, he could stay back at home to "practice" being home alone. He could eventually make this more challenging by extending the time he's alone and Anna is off doing errands and other activities.

Eventually Rafael will encounter a situation on his list that he'd never do without Anna. He'll need to break this task down into several steps so he gradually becomes more and more independent. Let's take something fairly concrete, like his refusal to go to the mall without Anna. Rafael could work on this dependency task by breaking it down into the following steps.

1.  Go to the mall with Anna and have her sit on a bench while he ventures alone into a nearby store, staying there for ten minutes. He does this repeatedly, each time extending the amount of time alone in the store beyond the initial ten-minute interval.

2.  Anna sits and has a coffee in the food court while Rafael ventures further into the mall, even temporarily losing sight of Anna. He does this repeatedly, each time going a little further into the mall.

3. Anna and Rafael shop separately, but since they both have cellphones, Rafael knows he can call Anna if needed.

4. Anna waits in the car while Rafael enters the mall alone.

5. Anna drops Rafael off at the mall and then leaves to do another errand.

There are situations on Rafael's list, like this one, that lend themselves very nicely to this graduated step-by-step approach; there are also other situations that are more difficult to do gradually. For example, you can either meet a friend for coffee or you don't. It's hard to imagine how you can gradually work yourself up to this task. Rafael waited on these activities until he built up his independence and confidence from conquering the more concrete situations on the list.

Rafael can expect to feel a surge of anxiety each time he takes the next step without Anna. In fact, it's important that Rafael feel some anxiety. Feeling the anxiety and navigating through it—rather than avoiding it—is the only way he can learn that he's not as anxiously helpless as he thinks. Ultimately, learning to deal with anxiety without Anna present will do wonders in rebuilding Rafael's self-confidence. His experience will teach him that he doesn't need Anna to get him through daily activities that others do so effortlessly.

## 3. Practice Taking Initiative

Before he began courageously addressing his anxiety, Rafael had been so demoralized by his dependency on Anna that he withdrew from sharing in the responsibilities and decision-making of family life. The anxiety had caused him to become risk aversive. He doubted his own judgment and was fearful of making mistakes. So Anna took full responsibility for parenting, finances, social activities, relations with their extended family, house repairs, and the like. Whenever she tried to include Rafael in decision-making, he simply walked away. He said he couldn't handle the stress; that it made him too anxious.

At a certain point, though, Rafael came to realize that rather than wait for full recovery from anxiety—he needed to work on reengaging with his family. And again, he started small and worked his way up, moving inch by inch out of his comfort zone and building his confidence gradually. He could start by getting involved in some minor decision-making, such as how to deal with the garden care and lawn mowing, what to do about snow removal in the winter, helping with meal planning, suggesting movies for the family to watch together, helping put the kids to bed, and the like. Rafael also realized that instead of withdrawing altogether, he could offer his opinion and then together with Anna make their decision. And as Rafael became more engaged in these minor responsibilities and decision-making, he graduated to more complex issues like their finances, whether to repair their car or buy new, and what to do about their daughter, who was falling behind in reading.

The final step in the process involved taking more initiative in some of the issues at home and work—like taking lead on the task of working with his daughter's school on a remedial reading plan. Of course, this greater involvement is risky, because taking control over problems means you could fail. But risk is a good antidote for fear and anxiety.

Anxious helplessness has effects far beyond how you deal with anxiety. If you believe you're emotionally weak and helpless, it affects how you work and relate to others, your level of intimacy and closeness to loved ones, and your involvement in parenting and household tasks. It can affect your motivation and interest in maintaining your fitness and physical health. If you believe, like Rafael did, that you're weak and vulnerable to anxiety, you'll start avoiding and become dependent on others. Not only will this confirm in your mind that you're weak, but others may begin treating you like an emotionally fragile person. Now you're caught in a vicious cycle that fuels your belief that anxiety is an insurmountable problem. That's why transforming your self-view from anxiously helpless to *anxiously capable* is such an important element of any strategy for overcoming anxious helplessness.

# What You Can Do

If you are caught in the vicious cycle of anxious helplessness, you'll want to use the three strategies covered in this chapter. There are a few other considerations when designing assignments based on these exercises:

- **Expect to feel anxious.** For an exercise to be effective, you need to feel at least some discomfort when challenging your sense of anxious helplessness. The goal is learning to tolerate anxiety and you can't improve your tolerance level if you don't experience anxiety.

- **Be systematic.** It's important to develop a plan for how you'll do the exercises over several weeks. For example, think ahead and write down the various steps you'll take to continue to challenge yourself over a four- to eight-week period.

- **Repeat, repeat, and repeat.** Repetition is the key to these exercises. If you try an assignment and it's overwhelming, don't give up. Think of ways to simplify it so you can work your way up to a more challenging assignment. Be patient and kind to yourself. And commit to keep going, even if it takes time and you encounter setbacks. Confronting our fears is hard work. So expect to feel drained after doing an assignment.

- **Self-reflection.** These exercises are about changing what you believe about your ability to tolerate anxiety. As you go, write down what your experience with these assignments indicates about your personality, strengths, and abilities. Are you discovering that you're emotionally stronger than you've been thinking? Are you more capable of handling anxiety than you realized? If your answer is "yes," to whatever degree, then you've dealt a serious blow to your belief in anxious helplessness.

# CHAPTER 5

# Catastrophizing

Catastrophizing: *a tendency to dwell on terrible worst-case outcomes that you're convinced could happen to you or your loved ones.*

What comes to your mind when you hear the word *catastrophe?* No doubt tragic life-changing events come to your mind—like floods, hurricanes, war, fatal motor vehicle accidents, or even the sudden, unexpected death of a loved one—events that make you feel like your world has collapsed and you'll never recover from it. Even more mysterious is another type of catastrophe that occurs only in our mind. We call it *catastrophizing* and for millions of people the anticipation of a possible catastrophe can be almost as distressing as coping with a real-life adversity.

Catastrophic thinking assumes that great calamity is just around the corner. If the doctor suggests more testing, the catastrophizer assumes it must be cancer. If a teenager is late coming home, the catastrophizer worries they are in great danger. If a partner has become more withdrawn, the catastrophic thinker can't stop thinking of possible infidelity. This was Debra's problem. Her habitual catastrophic thinking was driving her to a life filled with anxiety and worry. In this story you'll see all the elements that make catastrophic thinking a vicious cycle that's hard to break.

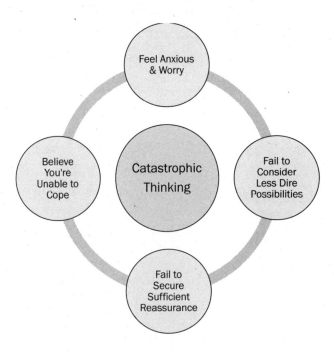

Figure 7

# Debra's Story

If asked to characterize her life in one sentence, Debra might respond, *Routine, predictable, and somewhat boring but also filled with fear and a terrible sense of foreboding.* This description seems contradictory, for how could life be rather routine and boring, devoid of crises or adversities, but also feel overwhelming and terrifying? Like others Debra faced the usual stresses and disappointments of daily living, but her life felt so much harder because of catastrophic thinking. Whatever the problem or difficulty, Debra always expected the worst. This was true of everything, from the small, routine tasks of everyday living to the really significant events in her life. When she went grocery shopping recently, for instance, Debra was convinced the store would be crowded and chaotic and the checkout lines exceptionally long— which would make her late once again for a doctor's appointment. She already was afraid her doctor was losing patience with her; what if he refused to see her again? Or the time something went wrong with the car. She was plagued by thoughts of the worst possible news, like having a huge repair bill or needing a part that was on backorder—and of their finances, already stretched thin. She absolutely needed the car for work! Speaking of work, recently there was talk of possible layoffs, and Debra was certain she'd be in the first round. She was in her early fifties, and the odds of finding new employment, she thought, were "slim to none." But the catastrophizing doesn't stop with external events. When it came to her health, Debra also imagined the worst. When experiencing an unexpected ache or pain, she worried it was due to a life-threatening disease like cancer. In every way Debra was a catastrophizer, and it was why she had chronic feelings of anxiety and worry.

Debra realizes her pessimism and negative thinking undermine her quality of life and relationships with others. She wants to be more positive and optimistic, but it just doesn't seem possible. Her mind automatically jumps to the most negative expectation. Predictions that the worst could happen feel more realistic, more likely to occur than a less negative outcome. They "feel right"—and anything less than the worst seems like brainwashing. Imagining the worst-case outcome also makes Debra feel anxious, which is all the proof she needs that the imagined catastrophe must be taken seriously. So, Debra spends a lot of time worrying, trying to prepare herself for the worst possible outcome.

Worst of all, Debra's "preparing for the worst" doesn't actually make her life easier. Her son is failing twelfth grade. He says he's bored and hates school. His attendance is spotty at best, and he refuses to do any homework. Last year his grades plummeted and this year it looks like he might not graduate. He's spending a lot of time with new friends. Debra worries about him incessantly. She's tried to talk to him about their "bad influence," but he doesn't listen. He just gets angry, yells at her, and storms out of the house. Debra's husband believes their son's just going through a phase, and he doesn't share Debra's concern. Debra has spent many sleepless nights worrying that her son will get mixed up in drugs and alcohol. Her catastrophic mind imagines him dropping out of high school, becoming ensnared in addiction, and ending up on the street in a state of hopeless despair. For Debra this catastrophic prediction is so real that it seems like a forgone conclusion. She is perpetually anxious and worried about her son, especially when he's defiant or disappears for several hours. The only time she feels relief from her worries is when he's home, but these occasions are becoming fewer with each passing day.

Debra's catastrophic thinking is "an albatross around her neck." It gives her a feeling of apprehension and sense of unease about the future. She's in a near constant state of anxiousness and relentless worry. It keeps her awake at night, she suffers from stomach aches and pains, and at times she has anxiety attacks when her worry peaks. She has difficulty dealing with present-day problems, like her son's school issues, because she is so preoccupied with what might happen. Her concentration at work suffers, she has become frightened to make decisions, and she often feels overwhelmed by the most trivial setback. All of this anxiety and worry stems from Debra's preoccupation with an uncertain future dominated by the possibility of some personal catastrophe that will change her life forever.

Does Debra's catastrophic thinking sound familiar? Do you get stuck in thoughts of a frightening future that only make you feel more anxious and worried? Maybe your catastrophizing focuses on a single issue like your health, finances, stability of your intimate relationship, or the welfare of your children. Or your catastrophizing may have spread such that you now imagine the worst for even routine daily activities and decisions. Whether you're a specific or generalized catastrophizer, there are several interventions you can use to counter catastrophic thinking and reduce anxiety and worry.

In the next section you'll see how Debra learned to treat imagined catastrophes as one of several possibilities and develop more confidence in her ability to deal with the most likely outcome to a difficult situation.

# How to Stop Catastrophizing

It's easy to slip into catastrophic thinking when you think it's helping you prepare for an uncertain future. But catastrophizing drives up anxiety so it's important to reverse this process. This can be done by learning to treat the imagined catastrophes as a possibility and not an inevitability, realizing that your catastrophic predictions most often are erroneous. This forces you to consider a more likely and less dire alternative.

## 1. Treat Thoughts as Thoughts Not Facts

Debra's work on breaking the catastrophizing habit begins with a profound realization that the *worst outcome* she imagines is a thought, a product of her mind, and not a fact about the future. It's an outcome that has not yet happened. It's still a possibility but not a reality. Just because the catastrophic thought feels like it will happen does not mean it will happen.

There's a simple strategy Debra used to shift her view of catastrophizing from *this is going to happen* to *I am thinking, imagining this could happen*. Every time she has the thought, *What if such and such happens?*, she replaces it with the phrase, *I'm having the thought that [insert catastrophe] could happen*. For example, when Debra thinks about her son's future, she pictures him wandering the streets as a drug-addicted, homeless adult. This image causes a spike in her anxiety, uncontrolled worry, and a profound feeling of helplessness. Instead, Debra can say to herself:

*I am having dark thoughts about my son. These are catastrophic thoughts that are just that, thoughts. I cannot know what the future holds for him. I suspect he'll have many struggles and difficulties. His life may start out more difficult than mine. I suppose my mind could create even worse outcomes than drug addict. I could imagine him committing some terrible crime like murder, becoming a terrorist, or a mass shooter. In fact, I have an active imagination and can even imagine flying elephants. Just because I can imagine flying elephants doesn't make them more real or likely to appear in the future. The same is true when I imagine a dark future for my son. There are many possible catastrophes I can imagine but they are all dark fantasy not reality. I'll treat them as thoughts ("flying elephants") and not facts.*

When Debra uses this self-talk strategy each time she catastrophizes, she's correcting her perspective on catastrophizing. She's reminding herself that catastrophic thoughts are just thoughts (one of several possibilities) and not inevitable facts.

## 2. Keep a Prediction Diary

In essence, catastrophizing is a prediction. It's looking into the future and thinking, *I'm convinced [insert catastrophe] is going to happen.* Debra constantly made dire predictions when something didn't go right. When she heard a rumor of possible layoffs at work, she predicted she'd be in the first round of cuts. When she was a few minutes late leaving the house, she felt anxiety build because she predicted traffic would be especially slow, she'd be hopelessly late for work, and she'd have to rush into an important early morning meeting all flustered and disorganized. When her manager called an unscheduled meeting, she found herself predicting she'd be in trouble.

Are you like Debra, always predicting the worst for yourself or loved ones? And have you ever considered how often your catastrophic predictions come true? The following exercise, called the *Prediction Diary*, is a good way to put your predictions to the test. (See http://www.newharbinger .com/53165 for the worksheet.) It goes like this: Debra begins by listing several significant problems, issues, or difficulties she's faced in the past. Next to each entry, she writes out the catastrophic prediction that made her anxious and worried. In a third column, she records the outcome—that is, what actually happened. As she completed the exercise, Debra realized she had no trouble thinking of numerous negative predictions she'd made recently—but she was surprised to learn that so few of those catastrophic predictions had actually come true. Instead, some alternative, far less negative outcome occurred. It got Debra thinking, *Why am I wasting my time on predictions that turn out to be so inaccurate?*

You can use this exercise to remind yourself that your catastrophic thinking is not an accurate prediction. But be careful when doing this exercise. Don't fall into the trap of trying to reassure yourself the catastrophe won't happen. Simply repeating to yourself, *This won't happen,* is not helpful, because none of us knows the future. Catastrophes do happen. The point of this exercise is to remind yourself that catastrophic thinking is not accurate; that catastrophizers tend to **overestimate the likelihood** that a catastrophe will happen, and a lot of time and mental effort can be wasted preparing for a catastrophe that never happens.

## 3. Think Outside the Box

Catastrophic thinking is like a runaway freight train; once you lose control, it's hard to stop. This happened to Debra when she started to feel anxious and worried about retirement. Saving for retirement was often on Debra's mind. She worried she and her husband were not putting enough away for retirement. Debra had lived through her parents' financial struggle in their senior years, and all she could imagine was reaching sixty-five with her and her husband's savings wiped out by poor investments and having to work well into her seventies.

To free herself from the trap of catastrophic thinking, Debra decides to use a *brainstorming exercise* to consider other possible outcomes associated with retirement. You can use the worksheet at http://www.newharbinger .com/53165.

Crucially, she works to think about a full range of possibilities, and not just the more positive ones. For example, Debra may have to work a couple of extra years; she may need to sell the house and move into an apartment to save money or rethink her "bucket list." (Notice these other options are negative but not as dire as the catastrophe.) Once the alternative list is generated, Debra reviews her list and considers which outcome is most likely. From there, whenever catastrophic thinking floods her mind, she can remind herself of the more likely outcomes.

Note this strategy can only work if you focus on more likely outcomes, even if they are not as desirable as you'd like. Often, people try to "think positively" when they worry, but this won't work. The most desirable outcome is often just as unlikely as the most catastrophic. In Debra's case, such outcomes might be: *We'll retire with lots of money due to wise investments, travel the world, vacation every winter in the sun, and enjoy excellent health well into our eighties.* But what she needs to do is focus on the most likely outcome— one that's quite possibly somewhat undesirable—and realize she can cope with that, even if catastrophizing has left her thinking she can't deal with anything that is undesirable.

## What You Can Do

Are you, like Debra, a catastrophizer? Do you get stuck on thinking the worst will happen when you're faced with challenges and difficulties? Does the worst possible outcome feel more real to you?

If your answer is "yes" to these questions, is it not time to change your anxious way of thinking? You can do this by following these steps.

1.  Make a list of all the current problems, issues, and situations that are the focus of your anxiety and worry. We'll call these your *anxious/worry concerns.*

2.  Briefly describe the catastrophic scenario associated with each concern. This is the worst possible outcome you're predicting for each concern.

3. Use the three intervention strategies that Debra used to dial down your catastrophic thinking bias.

4. Practice using these interventions each time you start to catastrophize. Remind yourself that the catastrophe is a thought, not reality. There are other negative outcomes that are more likely than the catastrophe, and you have coping skills to deal with these other outcomes. Like in the past, you will come through this difficulty better than you think.

Catastrophizing is another tough habit to break, especially if you're a chronic worrier. But the good news is that habits of the mind can be changed if you use the tools described in this chapter. But you will need to practice and be patient.

There is another anxiety process that makes catastrophic thinking more likely. Often, when thinking about the future fills you with anxiety, it's likely the unknowable is what bothers you most. If only you knew what was "just around the corner," you could be prepared. But you don't know, so you try to prepare for the worst. A tendency to catastrophize and an intolerance of uncertainty are the twin processes that accelerate anxiety about the future. As you read about uncertainty tolerance in the next chapter, consider working on both processes to reduce your anxiety and worry about the future.

# CHAPTER 6

# The Uncertainty Trap

Intolerance of uncertainty: *an inability to deal with the novel, ambiguous, or unpredictable without feeling intense anxiety or distress.*

If you had a choice, would you prefer to know immediately how a given situation turns out even if this increases the chance that the outcome will be undesirable, or would you prefer to live with the uncertainty of not knowing, because it increases the chance of a better outcome? Your answer to this question depends on whether you have high or low tolerance for uncertainty. Let's say you're invited to an interview for a highly desired job promotion. Would you prefer to know immediately that you didn't get the promotion, or would you like to wait two weeks for the interview committee to deliberate on your application? If your tolerance for uncertainty is low, you'd experience so much anxiety and worry from *not knowing* that you'd rather have the bad news now than wait for the possibility of a better outcome.

Why, you might ask, would someone rather face bad news now than wait for the possibility of better news in the future? As you'll see in the following illustration, there are several factors behind intolerance of uncertainty. If you have low tolerance for uncertainty, a novel, ambiguous, or unpredictable situation will be threatening and cause considerable anxiety. Your mind will race with "what if?" questions and none of the possibilities seem good. You're convinced you need to know what will happen right now because you can't cope with uncertainty. Your only way out of this anxiety trap is to seek safety in figuring out what is most likely to happen and then devising a plan to deal with it. Worry is the process of trying to prepare for possible future catastrophes. There is a strong connection between intolerance of uncertainty and worry.

You can see this connection between uncertainty intolerance and worry in Tierra's story. She has a strong need to know. Novel and unpredictable events cause an uncomfortable level of uncertainty that makes Tierra feel anxious and worried. But her world, like everyone's, is also filled with uncertainty, so she continually feels anxious and worried whenever she thinks about the future.

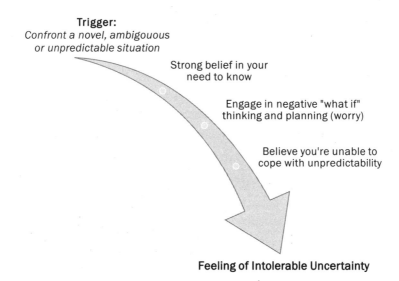

**Trigger:**
*Confront a novel, ambigouous
or unpredictable situation*

Strong belief in your
need to know

Engage in negative "what if"
thinking and planning (worry)

Believe you're unable to
cope with unpredictability

**Feeling of Intolerable Uncertainty**

Figure 8

# Tierra's Story

As a college-educated single woman employed in a lower-level clerical job, Tierra's life might seem boring and monotonous to many. Her parents believe she's fallen far short of her potential. But Tierra prefers things this way. She disdains adventure and embraces a life that is organized, structured, and predictable. She always plays it safe; she dislikes surprises and avoids taking risks as much as possible. She feels most comfortable when her days are planned, routine, and predictable, because of the anxiety and stress that emerge when the unexpected happens. The problem for Tierra is that life cannot be planned and predictable all the time. The unexpected can happen at any moment and the future is always uncertain. For this reason, anything that happens in the future causes Tierra anxiety. Her need to know coupled with an inability to tolerate uncertainty undermines her tranquility, plunging her into a heightened state of stress and anxiety because of her inability to deal with a future that could involve many "unknown unknowns."

Tierra's intolerance of uncertainty affects many important areas of her life. She has only a couple of close friends. Making new friends is too anxiety-provoking because she can never be certain they will accept her. She cannot risk the possibility of rejection. Besides, how can you know what people really think of you? She had a couple of serious intimate partner relationships but broke them off when she sensed they were getting serious. Tierra knows she has commitment issues that stem from uncertainty about her feelings and whether he was the right person for her. Because uncertainty is so distressing, a breakup seemed like the only solution to reduce the anxiety in her life.

Relationships aren't the only part of her life affected by uncertainty intolerance. Tierra was repeatedly encouraged to apply for promotions at work. Every time she turned down the opportunity because of a fear of the unknown. What if she couldn't do the job? What if she applied and was not successful? What if she accepted the promotion but then discovered it involved more responsibility, which might bring with it more scrutiny and less security? So Tierra decided to play it safe and stick with the job she knew so well.

Tierra's uncertainty intolerance affects even the more mundane, ordinary tasks of daily living. She always takes the same route to work, even if it is more congested. She rarely travels but when she does take a vacation she returns to the same resort year after year. Her diet is rather bland and monotonous because she doesn't like trying new food. And she shies away from movies that involve some level of suspense because she prefers predictable endings. Her choice of fashion hasn't changed in years, nor does she experiment with new hairstyles. She has lived in the same apartment for the past ten years and has little inclination to move or decorate it differently.

It should come as no surprise that Tierra finds decision-making especially painful. She often procrastinates, agonizing over the pros and cons of each possible option. But the endless analysis is rarely helpful, instead elevating her sense of uncertainty and heightening her anxiety and worry. Despite her desire to plan, Tierra is often gripped with worry about the future. As the years pass, her outlook on the future seems darker and more threatening. Anxiety and worry now dominate her day, as her fear of uncertainty intensifies.

Over the years, Tierra has come to the realization that her need for predictability is having a serious impact on her mental health. Fortunately for Tierra, there are strategies to learn greater tolerance of uncertainty. It begins with discovering you're probably more tolerant of uncertainty than you think and then systematically injecting more uncertainty into daily living.

## Boost Uncertainty Tolerance

Tierra's work on anxiety begins with realizing that the root of her problem is intolerance of uncertainty. If she can raise her level of uncertainty tolerance, reduce her need to know, and be less risk aversive, she'll be able to lower her anxiety and tendency to worry. There are three skills that Tierra needs to improve her tolerance of uncertainty: abandon efforts to attain a feeling of knowing what will happen in the future, strengthen her ability to accept novelty and change, and embrace the inevitability of uncertainty in daily living.

## 1. Confront the Illusion of Certainty

Uncertainty tolerance starts with realizing that the pursuit of absolute certainty is an impossibility because the future is inherently unknowable. For Tierra this means realizing that her attempts to attain a feeling of certainty are making her more rather than less anxious. What she is hoping to achieve is a feeling of knowing rather than some absolute fact or truth. This makes her pursuit of certainty even more tenuous because feelings are highly subjective and ephemeral. If she did attain her desired feeling of certainty, it would only last momentarily before being pulled back into doubt and uncertainty. Like anyone with anxiety due to low certainty tolerance, Tierra needs to work on altering her perspective in order to increase her certainty tolerance.

Keeping a Certainty Log is the first step in appreciating that uncertainty is not your enemy. See the worksheet at http://www.newharbinger .com/53165. Rather, accepting some level of risk and uncertainty is necessary for healthy living. Tierra can start by listing some common activities and decisions she makes without demanding a "feeling of certainty." For example, she drives to work each day without knowing she'll make it to her destination or whether the traffic will be heavier than normal. She uses online banking without a guarantee that she won't be hacked, and she buys groceries assuming the food is safe without knowing how it was manufactured. As Tierra lists the dozens of actions and decisions she makes every day without having perfect knowledge, she's surprised to learn her daily living requires considerable trust and acceptance that she'll be okay and life will go on. And, she thinks, if she can accept some uncertainty and not knowing outcomes in these situations, why not do the same in the new experiences and decisions that cause her so much anxiety and worry?

As Tierra reviews her list of uncertainty experiences, she learns that tolerance of uncertainty in these daily activities is evident because she believes in her ability to manage the situation and that a terrible outcome is highly unlikely. From the Certainty Log, it's clear Tierra has a baseline level of uncertainty tolerance and risk acceptance. So her goal is to increase uncertainty tolerance and apply it to the novel, more threatening experiences in her life. She can use the internal dialogue method to talk her way through feelings of uncertainty and anxiety about a new situation, like joining a gym. The dialogue might go like this:

> *Even thinking about joining a gym makes me anxious. I don't know what to expect but I know I do tolerate uncertainty in many things I do throughout the day. There's no reason I can't tolerate uncertainty about the gym as well. Of course, I can't know what will happen because I've never gone to a gym before. I've gotten through new experiences in the past and I can get through this one too. After all, what's the most likely negative outcome? Maybe no one will speak to me, which is just fine. In fact, I would prefer this to being the center of attention. Come on, Tierra, you can do this. Embrace your uncertainty and take this small risk.*

## 2. Novelty Inoculation

For Tierra making decisions and facing novel situations activates her uncertainty intolerance and subsequent anxiety. This means that building more novelty and decision-making into daily living is an important component in Tierra's work on raising her uncertainty tolerance.

This particular intervention is only effective if you start with fairly easy experiences of novelty and work up to more challenging situations. And for her part, Tierra found novelty so frightening that she needed to start her inoculation exercises with some fairly mundane changes in daily living. So she started with activities like taking different driving routes to work, eating at various new restaurants with cuisines she'd never tried before, inviting a friend to try out a new recreational activity with her, watching a few suspenseful movies, changing her hairstyle, and buying some new clothes. At first, she inevitably felt anxious about doing something novel, but the more she did it, the less distressing it became. And inevitably, as she took on novel experiences, she confronted her sense of uncertainty and learned to accept a higher level of not knowing.

As she became more comfortable with these minor changes, Tierra expanded her novelty inoculation to more intimidating experiences. For example, she agreed to apply for the next job promotion, plan a vacation to a new all-inclusive Caribbean resort, and create a profile for an online dating site. With each decision or new experience, Tierra confronted her uncertainty intolerance by writing down what more she'd need to know that would reduce risk and uncertainty. In most cases it was evident that she had all the knowledge necessary and a search for additional knowledge would not reduce the feeling of uncertainty.

Ultimately, with more new experiences under her belt, Tierra is learning to live a fuller, more interesting life with a better balance of risk and responsibility.

## 3. Tolerance Correction

Tierra's low tolerance for uncertainty, high need to know, and risk aversion causes her to feel anxious and worried whenever her mind drifts toward "what if" thinking about the future—but every occasion of anxiety or worry also presented her an opportunity to build greater tolerance for uncertainty. There's an exercise I call the *four-column tolerance tool* that Tierra used every time she felt anxious or worried to continue strengthening her tolerance capacity. (See http://www.newharbinger.com/53165 for the worksheet.)

The tolerance exercise starts with writing down the situation, problem, or circumstance that triggers an anxious feeling. For example, Tierra feels a wave of anxiety wash over her when she's reminded of the opportunity for a job promotion. As she begins working with the four-column tolerance tool, every time this happens, she writes it down. Next, she writes the best outcome she hopes to achieve in that situation—like hearing that she got the job promotion soon after applying for the position. In a third column, Tierra describes how she could make herself feel more certain that the best hoped-for outcome will occur—for instance, asking fellow coworkers whether they'd heard that others are applying for the promotion and whether management was desperate to fill the position.

The final step in this intervention is the most important: Tierra considers what she could do that is opposite to the ways to seek certainty that she wrote about in the third column. This task allows her to practice accepting a level of uncertainty that a less-than-desirable outcome might occur. That is, rather than trying to lower uncertainty by working to be convinced that a desirable outcome will occur, she does the opposite, which results in an acceptance of uncertainty. For Tierra, the opposite of seeking information from coworkers is not talking about the job position at work, reminding herself that she might not get the promotion, and that she has little control over the decisions of management. This forces Tierra to face the uncertainty of her promotion application. The more she practices the opposite of seeking certainty when feeling anxious, the more tolerant she'll become of feeling uncertain.

# What You Can Do

Maybe you're not sure whether low tolerance for uncertainty is an important feature of your anxiety and worry. If you feel anxious about making decisions or trying something new and unpredictable, then low uncertainty intolerance is probably driving up your anxiety. You'll want to spend extra time on the interventions described in this chapter to raise your tolerance level. But you'll need to be patient. Changing one's tolerance for feeling uncertain takes time and lots of practice because our level of comfort with uncertainty is linked to our personality. Think about the differences between a friend who is a thrill-seeker and loves the unexpected versus another friend who focuses on safety, predictability, and routine. One might love to go bungee jumping (thinking the cord might not hold produces an adrenaline rush), whereas the other might find flying a terrifying experience (thinking about the possibility of a plane crash produces panic). We all fall at different places on the spectrum between high and low tolerance of uncertainty.

Tolerance for uncertainty is also related to another anxiety process discussed in the next chapter, reassurance seeking. When tolerance for uncertainty is low, people often use reassurance seeking as a coping strategy to provide a false sense of knowing what will happen. So, know that the interventions you'll find in the reassurance seeking chapter will also be helpful in raising your uncertainty tolerance.

# CHAPTER 7

# Tell Me Again and Again

Excessive Reassurance Seeking: *repeatedly searching for or questioning people to obtain information or an opinion that agrees with your desired view that an anxiety-related situation is certain to be nonthreatening, benign, or safe.*

**Tell me what I want to hear!** Have you ever sought reassurance from a friend or family member hoping, even expecting, them to say what you want to hear? Suppose you're feeling anxious about the recent appearance of a skin rash. You're worried it could be skin cancer and so you make an appointment with the dermatologist. While waiting for the appointment, your anxiety builds. You ask your partner, "Do you think its nothing?" You're wanting your partner to say, "Oh, it's nothing. We all get skin rashes from time to time. It's normal." Seeking a desired answer or information is called reassurance seeking. Imagine how anxious you'd feel if your partner said, "How should I know? I'm not a doctor. I do recall a cousin who had a similar skin rash and it turned out to be melanoma." This comment would not be reassuring. It would drive up your anxiety to new heights.

Excessive reassurance seeking is a common feature of anxiety. It's the excessive and inappropriate use of a coping strategy familiar to all of us. How many times have you faced an important event in your life and turned to a friend, coworker, or family member and said, "Do you think it will be alright?" We want to hear the person say, "Oh I'm sure it will turn out fine." This is the answer you're looking for and it may bring momentary relief. If you think about it logically, though, it makes no sense, because our family member or friend can't predict the future. They don't know what will happen any better than you. So your mind has to do a magic trick to make the reassurance work. You have to believe that the more people you find that agree with your desired outcome (*It will be okay; you'll do fine*), the more likely it is that you'll get the desired outcome. You'll agree that phrased this way, this belief makes no sense. It's called an irrational belief. Even if a thousand people said it'll be fine, that will not increase the likelihood it will be fine. The only time their opinion might matter is when they are directly involved in the situation that concerns you—for example, when you're making a financial decision with your partner and you ask, "Are we making the right decision?" For the most part, they're as much in the dark about the future as you are!

It's also true that reassurance seeking is used to obtain temporary relief. For example, say you're feeling anxious and worried about a job interview scheduled for next week. You really need this job but your worry is interfering in your ability to prepare. You reach out to friends and family asking them, "Do you think I'll get the job? What if I'm so anxious that my mind goes blank and I can't answer questions? What if I have a panic attack and I'm sick to my stomach just before the interview?" You're hoping your friends will say, "You'll be fine. I'm sure you'll get the job even if you're feeling a little anxious. Everyone gets anxious during job interviews. You've done these interviews before and gotten the job." This is what you want your friends and family to say and for a moment you feel some relief. But before long you're having doubts about their reassurance, the outcome looks more uncertain, you start worrying again, and you're back to seeking more reassurance. When reassurance becomes a way of coping with anxiety and worry, it can easily become excessive. It becomes a vicious cycle as illustrated below.

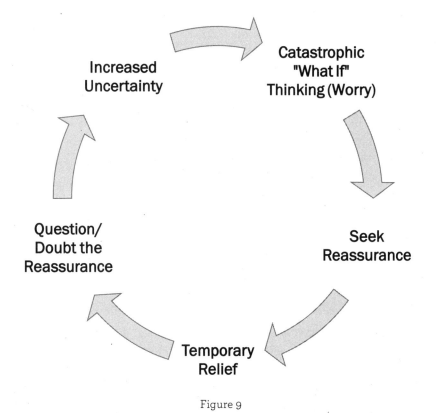

Figure 9

Take a look at Maya's reliance on reassurance to cope with her chronic worry. Her mind was stuck in "what if" thinking, causing her to search for information that would give her a sense that the worst would not happen.

## Maya's Story

Maya fretted about everything. She worried incessantly about any issue from the most mundane of daily activities like *What if I'm late leaving work and miss my aerobics class?* to more significant issues like *What if we run over budget again this month?* There was much to worry about in Maya's life. She was thirty-seven years old and beginning to notice a decline in her fitness level. She was starting a new job as a paralegal in one of the city's largest and most prestigious law firms. She and Sanjay had been together for fifteen years but lately their relationship had felt stale and routine. Maya worried they were drifting apart and wondered if Sanjay was seeing someone else. Their only child, twelve-year-old Jeong, was being bullied at school. Finances were also a concern. Before the COVID-19 pandemic, Maya and Sanjay moved into a larger house that required a hefty mortgage. Three years on with high inflation, the expenses of the new home were biting into their finances. There was little left over after paying all the bills, leaving them vulnerable if an unexpected expense arose.

Maya's life was fraught with many difficulties and problems but she felt paralyzed to do anything about them because of anxiety and worry. One of the strategies she used to deal with her distress was reassurance seeking. For example, she worried about Jeong's school difficulties. She met with his teacher several times but the meetings proved unhelpful. She kept asking Sanjay over and over whether he thought Jeong was frightened by the torment of his peers. In fact, she pestered Sanjay to the point where he sometimes became frustrated and angry, exclaiming, "What can I tell you so you'll stop haranguing me about Jeong?"

Maya searched the internet for information on bullying, but the suggestions never seemed practical or effective. She repeatedly questioned other mothers about their sons' school experiences, but it got her nowhere. In the end all these efforts to obtain reassurance proved futile, leading at most to temporary relief from her worry about Jeong. It was the same case at work. She was so scared of making a mistake that she'd repeatedly ask other paralegals to read her reports and evaluate their adequacy. The reassurance of one colleague was seldom enough; she'd ask two or even three people to read a report. Her requests were causing others to fall behind in their work and making her relationships with them tense. Eventually, Maya's manager had to intervene. But Maya still felt anxious and worried about her work, and she found herself compelled to ask her coworkers for verbal reassurance—which was less than satisfactory because the feelings of anxiety and worry quickly returned.

Several problems were evident with Maya's excessive reassurance seeking. It only brought her temporary relief from anxiety and worry. It reinforced a desire to avoid threat and uncertainty, and to embark on a relentless pursuit of safety. It contributed to a sense of personal responsibility and often it annoyed family, friends, and colleagues who could never say or do the right thing to relieve her anxiety. No matter what they said it was never good enough. Maya was caught in the vicious cycle of excessive reassurance seeking and it was making her more anxious and worried.

To break out of this self-defeating cycle Maya needed to change her perspective on reassurance seeking. She needed to fully understand its negative effects and its role in driving up her anxiety and worry rather than seeing it as a coping strategy or a way to find relief. Once she realized reassurance seeking was a way to manage feelings rather than a means of discovering a solution to the situations that caused her anxiety, she could then use strategies to gradually withdraw her reliance on this unhealthy coping strategy.

## Freedom from Reassurance

We all seek reassurance from time to time, especially when we're having doubts about a decision or course of action. But excessive reassurance seeking will drive up anxiety by instigating a vicious cycle of relief, doubt, and increased uncertainty. To break free of this unhealthy coping response, Maya needed to work on challenging her belief in the power of reassurance seeking, realizing the impossibility of obtaining perfect reassurance, gradually weaning herself off the reassurance seeking habit, and declaring to others that reassurance is being sought.

## 1. Changing Conviction

At the moment it happens, seeking reassurance seems like the best way to relieve anxiety and worry. To reduce her dependency on reassurance seeking, Maya first has to confront her belief in the power of reassurance. This involves discovering the futility of reassurance seeking, recognizing its negative impact, and realizing it's an accelerant of anxiety and worry. If she doesn't change how she thinks about needing reassurance, Maya will not stop seeking the advice and opinion of others.

There is a "tried and true" process for working on belief change. It starts with Maya writing down her experiences with reassurance seeking. She takes a blank sheet and creates three columns. (See http://www.newharbinger.com/53165 for the worksheet.) The first column head is "Reassurance About Threat," the second column heading is "Reassurance About Decisions," and the third column is "Reassurance About Social Acceptance/ Approval." Under the first column, she lists times when she felt intense anxiety or worry about the possibility of something terrible happening to her or a loved one, and she sought reassurance that everything will turn out fine. In the second column Maya writes down times she sought reassurance that she made the right decision on some important issues in her life. In the final column she records times when she sought reassurance about being loved, approved, or accepted by family or friends.

Hardly a day passed without Maya asking for reassurance, so she needed to list only the most significant experiences that stood out in her mind. The following illustrates some of Maya's reassurance seeking experiences.

## Reassurance About Threat

- Had to fly alone for first time; kept asking friends whether I'd be okay or whether I might get confused, upset, and become so anxious that I missed my flight.

- When I was in school, I was so anxious before tests; I was always asking my parents if I'd do okay or be so anxious that my mind went blank.

- Received notice that I needed a repeat mammogram; terrified I had breast cancer; kept asking my mother and Sanjay whether they thought the retest would be negative; also kept looking up information online.

## Reassurance About Decisions

- Thinking about going back to school for paralegal training; kept asking people whether or not this was the right decision for me.

- Was unsure of the best school for Jeong; kept asking other parents for their opinion of different schools; spent hours researching online.

- When Sanjay proposed, I accepted but then was tormented with doubts about my decision; talked endlessly to my mother and close friends about whether Sanjay was the "one" for me.

## Reassurance About Social Approval/Acceptance

- Working on my Facebook page; concerned what other people are thinking; repeatedly asked friends and family whether they liked the changes or not; kept seeking their honest opinion.

- Worried about our marriage; keep asking Sanjay if he still loves me.

- My mother and I were always very close, but I've noticed she seems less interested in me and my life the last couple of years; I keep asking her what's wrong and she says nothing's wrong.

In the final step of belief restructuring, Maya reviewed the reassurance seeking experiences she listed and answered the following questions.

- Was reassurance seeking helpful in any way? Did it contribute to a significant reduction in anxiety and worry?

- Did the reassurance provide any lasting sense of safety, security, or comfort?

- Were there any negative consequences associated with excessive reassurance seeking? Did it really solve anything? Did it contribute to a persistence of anxiety and worry? Did it seem to annoy people? How did other people react to the reassurance requests?

After doing this exercise, Maya's view of reassurance seeking changed. Rather than thinking of it as a helpful coping strategy, she found that her reassurance seeking was largely detrimental and an important contributor to her anxiety and worry. And she was then ready to use the next three interventions to change her approach to excessive reassurance seeking.

## 2. Define Your Perfect Reassurance

Reassurance is never perfect. When we ask people if they think it'll be okay, we already know their answer has no validity because they don't know the future any more than we do. But we keep on asking anyway. That's why whatever we're told, it never completely eliminates anxiety or worry. But few of us stop to realize the impossibly high standard any reassurance would have to meet to eliminate our anxiety and worry. That's why this next exercise can be helpful in reducing excessive reassurance seeking.

Maya can start the exercise by considering each of her worry concerns. She then writes out what she imagined would be perfect reassurance for each concern. This would be reassurance that would stop her anxiety and worry dead in their tracks. She wrote the following.

- If a teacher told me that Jeong had several school friends and she knew that no one would dare bully him now, then I'd stop worrying.

- If someone could convince me Sanjay would never have an affair, that he was not capable of cheating, I'd stop feeling so insecure about our relationship.

- I'd never worry about the quality of my work if the senior law partners told me I was an unbelievably talented paralegal, that they could never exist without me, and that my work was always impeccable.

- I'd never be anxious about finances if someone said they knew we'd always meet our financial obligations and would be able to save plenty of money for a comfortable retirement.

Maya concluded from a review of her list that perfect reassurance was impossible. Any "real-world reassurance" would fall far short of this "perfect reassurance" so it would be unable to eliminate her anxiety and worry. If this is true, then why bother continuing to seek fallible reassurance from others? Better to cut down on a strategy that promised so little and only made anxiety worse.

## 3. Delay Tactic

Excessive reassurance seeking is a difficult habit to break because it happens so quickly, without much thought or effort. This was true for Maya, so she needed to wean herself off it gradually. She did this by systematically lengthening the time between feeling anxious or worried about something and then asking for someone's opinion or searching for reassuring information. For example, Maya has the thought *Sanjay seems so withdrawn and distant* and then feels anxious about the relationship. Normally within five minutes she's talking to Sanjay about their marriage and his feelings, trying to be reassured of his love and commitment. Rather than trying to stop "cold turkey," Maya decides to sit with her anxiety for ten minutes before speaking to Sanjay. After a week or two, she extends the delay to twenty minutes, and then a half hour, working up to a two-hour delay. Once she reaches that level, the anxiety has dropped off and she is able to suppress reassurance seeking completely. By taking this approach to each of her anxious concerns, Maya could cut excessive reassurance seeking from her life.

## 4. Declare Reassurance Seeking

This next intervention requires considerable courage but it's very effective in countering the perceived benefits of reassurance seeking. What do you think would happen if Maya told people exactly what she wanted to hear them say when she sought reassurance? Take her anxiety about Sanjay having an affair. Normally, Maya sought reassurance by looking for indications that Sanjay loves her and is committed to the marriage. But any reassuring signals she got from him didn't reduce her anxiety or worry. So what if she said to Sanjay:

*I want to hear you say you're not having an affair, that you'll never cheat on me, and that you are completely committed to our relationship and that will never change as long as I live. Also, you have to say this with such deep conviction that I believe with absolute certainty that you'd never leave me no matter what happens.*

Of course, this would be a difficult and potentially embarrassing admission to make. Sanjay would never be able to make such a statement if he were honest. The future is unknowable. The only guarantee is the future will be different from what we imagine today.

By declaring her ideal reassurance (what she wants to hear), Maya is further reducing the power of reassurance seeking. It becomes quite useless to continue to seek reassuring signals from Sanjay now that they both know what she really wants to hear. It makes it hard to keep up the "charade" of reassurance seeking. Of course, this strategy can only be used with friends or family members with whom you have a close and honest relationship.

## What You Can Do

Have you decided that reassurance seeking is contributing to your anxiety and worry? If so, consider using some of Maya's interventions to break free of your dependency on these unhealthy coping strategies. I have some suggestions you might consider when trying to reduce excessive reassurance seeking.

- Start with the first two interventions and spend extra time with them. Most of us tend to think reassurance seeking is not harmful. You'll need to be convinced that reassurance seeking is an important contributor to your anxiety or worry to be motivated to change. The first two interventions focus on discovering the problem with excessive reassurance seeking.

- If you have difficulty recalling reassurance experiences in the first exercise, try keeping track of these experiences over a two- or three-week period. You'll find it more helpful if you categorize them as reassurance about threat, reassurance about decisions, or reassurance about social approval/acceptance.

- Be careful using the fourth intervention. Too much self-disclosure to people you can't trust could be detrimental. Use this strategy only with people you are close to and can be completely honest with. It may be embarrassing to admit what reassuring message you really want to hear even with your most intimate and trustworthy family and friends. But if you can do it, declaring your reassurance desires cancels out the benefits of this unhealthy coping strategy. This is because both you and your reassurer know the game is up on providing reassurance to ease your anxiety or worry.

- Have you considered the effect your excessive reassurance seeking has on family, friends, and coworkers? Most people find repeated reassurance seeking annoying because whatever they say, it's not good enough. Realizing the negative effect excessive reassurance seeking is having on your relationships can boost your motivation to change.

Reassurance seeking is a tough habit to break because we do it without even thinking. It's also a coping strategy related to many of the processes that fuel anxiety and worry. The next chapter considers one of these processes, inflated responsibility. When you incorrectly assume you might be responsible for some unfortunate circumstance happening to you or a significant person in your life, you're more likely to seek relief in the reassurance of others.

# CHAPTER 8

# It's All My Fault

Inflated responsibility: *believing you have a significant impact in causing or preventing negative experiences happening to you or others. Whether these negative experiences are events that might happen, or they are actual events that already happened, you believe there is a moral consequence to your action or inaction.*

Are you guilt-ridden? When anxious or worried, do you often feel responsible for doing something that caused a negative outcome or not doing something that could have prevented it? If so, you may have an inflated sense of responsibility that drives up self-blame so you are often flooded with feelings of guilt.

Let's say you're late for work on a day you were scheduled to make the introductory remarks for a team presentation. Everyone in the meeting is waiting for you. You're feeling anxious knowing you're responsible for holding up the meeting. And you feel guilty because you've violated a personal moral imperative to be on time. This is an example of a normal, healthy sense of responsibility.

But what if you feel responsible for causing or preventing negative events over which you have little influence or control? Your coworker's team presentation is poor and you blame yourself for not coaching him, your partner has a flat tire and you think you should have checked the tires that morning before going to work, your child does poorly on a test and you think it's your fault for not doing extra homework with her, the credit card bill is too high but you blame yourself even though your partner places online orders daily, or you see a nail in the street and then think you could have prevented an accident by picking it up. You probably agree that these are examples of inflated or unreasonable responsibility. Can you see how a person who overestimates their responsibility in so many daily activities would tend to feel more anxious and worried? Having an inflated sense of responsibility also makes you feel guilty—an emotion that can fuel anxiety and worry.

As you'll see in the next story, Carlos had an excessive sense of personal responsibility that caused him to feel anxious, worried, and guilty more often than not.

## Carlos's Story

Sorry could be Carlos's middle name. He apologizes for every mishap, big or small, that happens at home or at work. It doesn't matter what it was, whether he was directly involved or not, Carlos feels responsible and apologizes. From the most obvious, like forgetting to answer an email, to the most unlikely, like a coworker missing a deadline, Carlos imagines some reason he'd be responsible for causing the unfortunate event, or not preventing it. Because of his excessive sense of personal responsibility, Carlos lives in a perpetual state of self-blame and guilt. This contributes to a broader feeling of apprehension and worry that something unfortunate was imminent and he'd be held responsible.

Carlos reacts more strongly than most to actions and decisions for which we'd all feel some degree of moral responsibility. Not being truthful, taking credit when not deserved, covering up a mistake, saying something rude or offensive, or being pushy with others are examples of normal situations associated with a sense of personal responsibility and guilt. But Carlos feels anxious and guilt-ridden for weeks after a moral violation, even when often, the consequence is negligible even to the person offended. And then there are other experiences that have little to do with Carlos and yet he assigns himself undue responsibility for these outcomes. In these instances of "irrational responsibility," Carlos hears of a mishap and then searches for connections to it that make him responsible for causing or not preventing the mishap.

For instance, Carlos works on a team that is responsible for preparing stock market forecasts for senior management. These analyses are crucial because investment decisions are made based on the forecasts. All forecasts are made by consensus in the team. In a volatile stock market, the team's forecasts could be off. Often, when this happens, Carlos takes all the blame. He feels he should have known how the market would react and he should have warned his team members. Overwhelmed with guilt, he starts apologizing to his team and even senior management for not making better market predictions. He believes it's his fault that the firm loses money on some of its investments. In reality, even a renowned investor like Warren Buffet can't possibly foresee all the ups and downs in a turbulent stock market. And Carlos is on a team; he doesn't have sole responsibility for the decisions they make. All this self-blame and guilt, fed by an inflated sense of personal responsibility, only heightens Carlos's anxiety and worry about producing the next market forecast.

Carlos's inflated responsibility is also evident at home. His wife has a flat tire on the way to work. She immediately calls him in a panic because she'll miss an important meeting. She's clearly flustered and upset. *I should've checked the tire pressure before she left,* he thinks, and a wave of intense guilt washes over him. But of course, there was no reason to believe his wife would have a flat tire. How could he have anticipated that she would? In another example Carlos's coworker comes to work one day and reports that she rear-ended a car while at a traffic intersection; Carlos blames himself for not warning her about the dangers of texting and driving. And then there is Carlos's father-in-law. He recently fell off a ladder while fixing an eaves-trough, fracturing his hip, and now requires hip surgery. Carlos feels guilty. He mentioned to his father-in-law that he should stay off ladders, but now he thinks he should have gone further and taken the ladder away, and fixed the eavestrough himself.

There are several factors that drive the anxiety and worry associated with inflated responsibility.

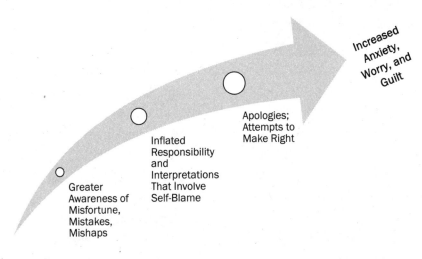

Figure 10

We live in a world where mishaps and misfortune can happen to anyone at any time. If you overthink personal responsibility, you'll feel on edge waiting for "the other shoe to drop." As you see in the previous figure, you'll start by being more tuned in to mishaps and misfortunes in your personal world. When misfortune strikes, you'll immediately consider your level of responsibility and blame. You'll try to correct your perceived wrongdoing by an apology or trying to put things right. In this way your inflated sense of personal responsibility keeps you in a state of anxiety and worry over what negative incident will happen next.

# Recalibrate Inflated Responsibility

For Carlos to ease his anxiety and guilt, he needs to develop a more balanced, rational perspective on moral responsibility. He has a distorted view of his control over events, so he first has to gain a greater appreciation of the multitude of influences that cause a mishap. Then he can use an inductive reasoning technique to realize the impossibility of preventing a misfortune. He can then practice thinking of personal responsibility as a continuum of increasing degrees of responsibility for the negative experiences in his life. By practicing these strategies whenever he felt anxious and guilty, Carlos will be able to dial back on excessive responsibility and self-blame.

## 1. The Responsibility Pie

At the root of inflated responsibility is a misunderstanding of influence and control. Carlos believes he has influence over events that are really outside his control. When he felt guilty for not warning his colleague about the dangers of texting and driving, he had to be convinced that she'd heed his warning and stop texting, that he had the power to stop her from texting while driving. Does he really? Isn't she an adult who'll decide how she drives? No doubt Carlos's coworker already knew not to text while driving, so hearing a lecture from Carlos would only annoy her. It might even cause strained relations in the office. Carlos was assuming way too much influence over his coworker; he assumes the same in a lot of his relationships. So, his work on inflated responsibility starts by addressing his exaggerated sense of influence and control over bad outcomes. He did this by completing a responsibility pie chart. (See http://www.newharbinger.com/53165 for the worksheet.)

Let's take a different problem, Carlos thinking he should have prevented his father-in-law from falling off a ladder. Start the exercise by listing all the factors that went into causing the misfortune that is bothering you. You can see Carlos's list below.

| Possible Causes of the Fall | % Contribution to Cause of the Fall |
|---|---|
| Father-in-law's decision to use the ladder | 40% |
| Father-in-law has a dizzy spell while on the ladder | 20% |
| Used an old ladder | 3% |
| Ladder poorly positioned against the house | 5% |
| Mother-in-law was home but didn't know he was on ladder | 10% |
| Wife didn't get around to talking to her father about using ladders given his poor balance | 16% |
| The weather: it had rained the night before and everything was slippery | 5% |
| I [Carlos] should have stopped my father-in-law using the ladder | 1% |

The next step in the exercise is the most difficult. As you'll see from Carlos's example, in the second column, you'll write down an estimate of what percent each factor played in causing the misfortune. For Carlos that meant thinking deeply about all the causes that contributed to his father-in-law's fall and estimating how important each was in causing the fall. The percentages had to add up to 100 percent and Carlos needed to estimate his contribution last. Also, Carlos had to base his estimates on reason and logic, not on his feelings. Naturally, he had to admit that his father-in-law's decision to use the ladder, and then the fact that he had a dizzy spell while on it, contributed most to causing the fall. He also gave his wife a fairly high rating because she had special influence over him, as his child; she should have said something to her father about staying off ladders. But notice that by the time Carlos got to himself at the end of the list, there was only 1 percent left. Carlos may have felt like he had 40 percent responsibility for the fall, but in reality, he had only 1 percent influence at most.

It's often helpful to create a picture of these various contributions in the form of a pie chart. From his responsibility pie chart, Carlos is able to see that he had only a sliver of influence over preventing his father-in-law's fall. And if you have little influence over an event, how can you blame yourself for the misfortune? Having a more realistic perspective on your influence over a bad outcome is the first step toward correcting the inflated responsibility bias.

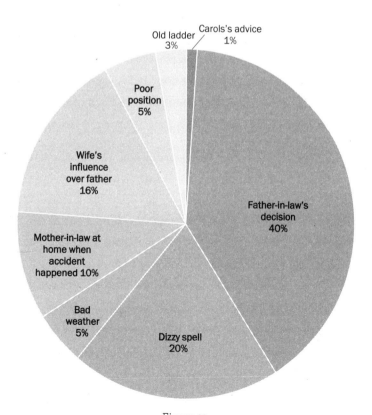

Figure 11

## 2. Think It Through

Often emotions seem to occur without reason. When this happens—we call them irrational and this often happens with issues of control, responsibility, and morality. Once you feel responsible for causing or not preventing misfortune, you might automatically assume it's true. The anxiety and guilt reinforce your belief that you have influence over the negative outcome because why else are you feeling so bad about it. This is exactly what happened to Carlos. He got caught into the inflated responsibility trap without ever stopping to think it through; to ask himself whether it was even possible to prevent a particular misfortune. Because he felt anxious and guilty, he just assumed he was justified in thinking he was responsible in some way.

The next exercise helps counter inflated responsibility by training your mind to think more deeply about your actual influence and connections to unfortunate events. Take Carlos's feeling of responsibility for not preventing his wife's flat tire. The car was only a year old and the tires were hardly worn. It was a clear spring morning, so the driving conditions were excellent. How could Carlos possibly know that today his wife would have a flat tire? Using the "think it through" exercise, Carlos wrote out how he'd have to think irrationally about the flat tire incident to justify feeling responsible for preventing it.

> It's my responsibility to ensure that both our vehicles are in good working order. I should have checked the tire pressure on all four tires before my wife left for work. I should do that every day of my life. I should have felt each tire to ensure there were no punctures. If I did this each morning, it would be impossible for my wife to have a flat tire. The only reason flat tires occur is because of low tire pressure, an existing puncture, or some visible weakness in the tire. Flats can't be caused by running over sharp objects on the road or hitting a large pothole. As the driver of the vehicle, my wife holds no influence on whether she has a flat tire. I am the sole person that has influence over the tires, whether they stay inflated or lose air.

As Carlos reviewed what he wrote, he could see many false statements. Low tire pressure is not the main cause of a flat; running over a sharp object is a much more likely cause, and there's no way to prevent that from happening. It's totally unreasonable to check tire pressure every time you drive a car, and even that wouldn't guarantee you'd get no flats. Carlos was able to see that his self-blame for the flat tire was totally unreasonable. It was based on faulty reasoning. If his reasoning is faulty, then his inflated responsibility estimates were faulty as well.

## 3. The Responsibility Continuum

By now you might be thinking, *Surely not all responsibility is misguided or inflated.* We all have some influence over what happens in life, and there are times we do bear responsibility for causing or not preventing misfortune to ourselves or others. At times it can be difficult to know whether our sense of responsibility is reasonable or whether it's exaggerated and causing unhealthy anxiety and guilt. Consider the case of a young man who jumped onto the tracks of an approaching subway to save a woman who fell on the track because of a heart attack. He saved the woman and lived to tell the tale. Did he have an unreasonable or admirable sense of responsibility for saving the woman's life? Sometimes it can be difficult to know what is healthy and what is unhealthy responsibility. This was Carlos's dilemma. Because he felt responsible for so many things that happened, he'd lost the ability to distinguish between normal responsibility and excessive or inflated responsibility.

The responsibility continuum can help you recalibrate your responsibility estimates so they are more realistic and less toxic for anxiety and guilt. (See http://www.newharbinger.com/53165 for the worksheet.) It starts by thinking of personal responsibility as a continuum that runs from 0 percent responsibility at one end to 50 percent responsibility in the middle and then 100 percent responsibility at the other end. Next list four to five experiences for each of the three levels of responsibility. Take a look at Carlos's continuum as an example.

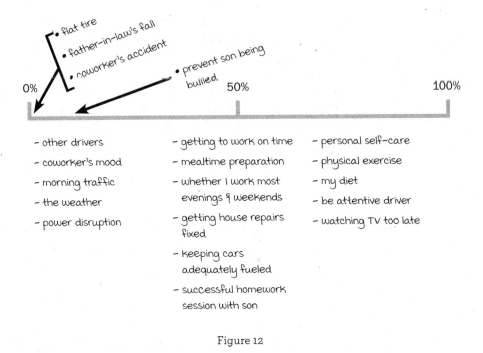

Figure 12

Carlos discovered that many of his daily experiences revolved around the 50 percent mark. He had some influence and responsibility over these experiences but it was far from complete. Others also had considerable influence in causing or preventing these occurrences.

The final step in the continuum exercise is to review the experiences associated with your inflated responsibility estimates and place them on the continuum. This is the most important part of the exercise. When Carlos re-examined his responsibility estimates, he realized most of them were very close to 0 percent responsibility compared to everything else happening in his life. He placed "preventing his son from being bullied" a little higher because he thought he should take initiative and enroll his son in a self-defense course.

Carlos found the responsibility continuum especially helpful in dialing back his inflated responsibility. He realized he was spending far too much time on things with near zero responsibility to the detriment of the many experiences in life where he had 50 percent or higher influence and responsibility. He resolved to focus more attention on these higher responsibility experiences and "let go" of the low responsibility events where there was little or no possibility of influencing the outcome.

# What You Can Do

If self-blame and guilt play a role in your anxiety, then inflated responsibility is probably a problem you'll want to tackle. As you can see from the interventions in this chapter, working on inflated responsibility requires a change in how you see your influence and control over events in your life. If you decide to use these exercises to free yourself from the inflated responsibility trap, let me offer three suggestions.

- Make sure you focus on instances of inflated, exaggerated, and faulty responsibility. These are times when you overthink your responsibility for mishaps that you have little influence on causing or preventing. If you find the exercises unhelpful, maybe you're focused on an experience of legitimate responsibility. For instance, you take your car in for an oil change and the technician advises that you need a brake job. You ignore his advice because new brakes would be expensive. Later your teenage daughter has a traffic accident because the brakes failed. In this case you share much of the responsibility for this misfortune because you could have prevented it. There's nothing to work on in this case because you should feel responsible.

- Don't get stuck in your emotions. Just because you feel guilty doesn't mean your responsibility estimate is accurate. Stick to what the exercises are telling you. Do they indicate that your responsibility estimate is inaccurate and excessive because you have little influence over causing or preventing a misfortune?

- Use these exercises repeatedly over many different types of relevant experiences. With time and practice you'll become more skilled at correcting the faulty attributions of responsibility that fuel your anxiety and guilt. You can also ask your partner, close friend, or therapist to help with the exercises. Sometimes the perspective of another person can be helpful when you're stuck in your own biased and limited understanding of a situation.

With inflated responsibility, anxiety arises because you overestimate how much influence and control you have over negative experiences. But personal responsibility is not the only way beliefs about control can cause anxiety. Beliefs about the potential for uncontrollability can also drive up anxiety. This is the subject of our next chapter.

# CHAPTER 9

# Could I Snap?

Fear of losing control: *a belief in the possibility of being overwhelmed by negative emotion that results in a loss of voluntary control over thoughts, feelings, or behavior that would cause embarrassment, distress, or harm to self or others.*

Have you ever thought, *I think I'm losing my mind?* Maybe this occurred when you felt completely overwhelmed because so many things were coming at you, and you couldn't handle any more bad news. And then you got more bad news and you thought, *I can't take it; I'm going to snap.*

"Snap" is an interesting word. We think of a rope snapping when there's too much pressure and it breaks in two. When the word is applied to our mind and we think of our mental health "snapping," its meaning is less clear. Do you think of it as stress or mental pressure building inside to the point that you feel a surge of negative emotion or distress? Does the anxiety, frustration, anger, guilt, or some combination of these emotions become so intense that you fear the possibility of losing control altogether?

People have different ideas of what it means to "lose mental control." For some it's a loss of emotional control in which they start screaming, yelling, or showing intense displays of emotion that cause embarrassment, shame, or humiliation. For others it's a loss of control over their behavior where they may become rude, offensive, or maybe even aggressive. Some people consider a panic attack a form of "snapping," whereas for others it's suddenly bolting from an uncomfortable situation. Whatever you envision, a common feature is *perceived loss of control.* Many people with anxiety live in a constant fear of losing control.

There are several processes that maintain a fear of losing control.

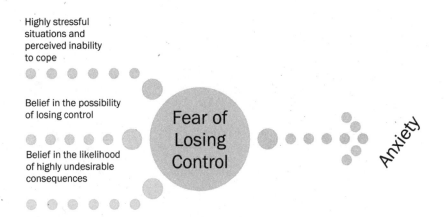

Figure 13

Before we continue, it's important to distinguish fear of losing control from actual loss of control. It's all too common to see people lose control, usually in the form of anger, aggression, rude and offensive comments, or inappropriate displays of emotion. Some people have poor impulse control that can cause grievous harm to self and others. If you have anger management issues or poor impulse control, I encourage you to seek professional help given the likelihood you're causing significant harm to yourself, family, coworkers, friends, and maybe even strangers.

This chapter is about fear of losing control. It's written for people who have reasonably good self-control but fear the possibility of losing control. If this describes you, you may feel anxious because of doubt and uncertainty that you can trust your self-control over unwanted thoughts, feelings, and behavior. It's a lack of confidence in your level of self-control. As you see from the diagram above, a fear of losing control involves several factors like seeing your circumstances as highly stressful and beyond your capacity to cope with, believing that you could lose control, and imagining highly undesirable consequences if you snapped.

As you'll learn from her story, the fear of losing control is a root cause of Amber's anxiety, and it greatly limited the effectiveness of her therapy.

## Amber's Story

Amber, a single adult in her early thirties, has a permanent job in retail that gives her a degree of independence and financial stability. Growing up in a low-income, single-parent family, she was forced to assume greater responsibility for her younger brother and sister than would be expected for her age. Now one of the lasting effects of her childhood is an abiding fear of losing control. Amber has become a very controlled person. She finds it impossible to be spontaneous, preferring instead to have everything planned out in a predictable manner. Those who know her find her serious, deliberate, disciplined, and yes, humorless. Amber feels most comfortable when she's in control. The unexpected, novel, and ambiguous are especially challenging for her.

Many experiences cause Amber to feel anxious because of her fear of losing control. Once when crossing a high multilane suspension bridge over the Hudson River, Amber had the impulse to suddenly veer the car toward the side of the bridge. She imagined the car jumping over the guard rail and plunging 200 feet into the river below. The image was so vivid and the emotion so powerful that Amber developed a fear of driving across suspension bridges. What, she wondered, did these terrifying thoughts mean? Did losing control of the thoughts mean she had poor self-control—and that she might act on those thoughts someday?

In another example Amber had the intrusive impulse of jumping in front of an approaching bus or delivery truck while standing at a pedestrian crosswalk. The impulse scared her so much that she refused to stand close to the curb. The same impulse popped into her mind when waiting for a train or subway, so again she stood well back from the edge of the platform. Amber wondered if these unwanted impulses meant she had some type of unconscious death wish and that, in time, her mind would eventually snap and she'd try to kill herself.

Amber also had unwanted intrusive thoughts of a sexual nature that caused her great anxiety. One evening she was visiting a friend and her four-year-old daughter wanted Amber to read stories to her. As Amber started to read, the thought *Am I becoming sexually aroused by having Katie sit on my lap?* popped into her mind. The intrusive thought was extremely upsetting, so Amber immediately started scanning her body for signs of sexual arousal. She thought she felt a twitch in her inner thighs and wondered if she was getting aroused. This was a horrifying prospect because Amber took it as a sign she might be a "latent pedophile." Was she capable of losing control and actually harming a child? The fear of losing control, and perpetrating an unspeakable crime, caused Amber such anxiety around children that she avoided them as much as possible. She could not even watch TV shows or movies that included children because she feared the sight of little girls, in particular, might elicit unwanted, disgusting thoughts and feelings.

Although Amber feared losing control, she actually was a highly controlled, moral person. Honesty and integrity were core values she lived by. Anyone who knew Amber considered her stable, controlled, and reliable.

She rarely showed strong or uncontrollable emotion, was planned, structured, and deliberate in her actions, and always took time to think about how to respond to others. If anything, family and friends were inclined to characterize Amber as overly controlled. Her friends would often say, "Amber, you need to loosen up, girl, be less serious and have some fun." Little did they know that Amber was gripped by a fear of losing control. Contrary to their beliefs, Amber was convinced her problem was too little control rather than too much control.

Does Amber's experience with control sound familiar to you? Are you afraid of losing mental control; that you'll snap and do something embarrassing or harmful? Are there things you avoid because of a fear of losing control? If this is your story, consider how Amber worked on building trust in her self-control and became more comfortable with spontaneity.

## Testing the Limits

To overcome this fear, Amber needed to build trust in her ability to control her thoughts, feelings, and behavior. She did this by learning that self-control is a matter of degree, that she's never lost complete self-control and suffered serious negative consequences, and that her greater problem is too much rather than too little self-control. She also learned to harness spontaneity in countering her control fears.

### 1. Close to the Brink

How close have you come to snapping? I don't mean the feeling or fear of snapping but acting in a way that was out of character because of a complete loss of control. Also, I'm not talking about doing something funny, or silly, or even taking a chance. I'm thinking of an incident involving a serious consequence where you acted on pure impulse without regard to yourself or others. What is the closest you've come to a complete loss of control?

Amber started work on her fear of losing control by thinking of self-control as a continuum in which she has different degrees of self-control depending on the circumstance. At one end she described what she imagines an absolute lack of self-control would involve. This would be 0 percent self-control. Then she described what the other end of the continuum would be, that is, 100 percent absolute self-control over thought, feeling, and action. This is Amber's view on the extremes of self-control.

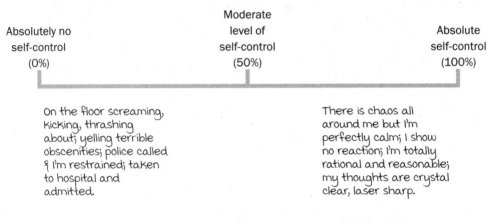

Moderate
level of
self-control
(50%)

Absolutely no
self-control
(0%)

Absolute
self-control
(100%)

On the floor screaming, kicking, thrashing about; yelling terrible obscenities; police called & I'm restrained; taken to hospital and admitted.

There is chaos all around me but I'm perfectly calm; I show no reaction; I'm totally rational and reasonable; my thoughts are crystal clear, laser sharp.

Figure 14

Next, Amber plots all her experiences involving a fear of losing control on the continuum. (See http://www.newharbinger.com/53165 for the worksheet.) For instance, she has an unwanted, horrific intrusive thought that she's sexually attracted to children. Where would she place that experience on the self-control continuum? Certainly, it is more than 0 percent self-control because she's never harmed a child, not even come close. But self-control is also not 100 percent because the disgusting sexual thought popped into her mind against her will. So maybe she concludes she has 60 percent self-control. Is there really anything to fear when you have that level of control over thoughts, feeling, and behavior? After all, it would be the experiences close to 0 percent that you might fear losing control over. All the rest involve sufficient self-control to prevent a truly dreadful consequence.

There is one final step in this exercise. Amber then recalls the very worst experience of losing self-control. (It was when she was young—a time her younger brother had snuck out of school and didn't come home, forcing Amber to go and look for him. When she finally found him, Amber recalled, she'd lost it completely. She started screaming at him and crying for being "so stupid." She was terrified he had gotten into trouble and was in police custody.) Even in this situation Amber had 20 percent self-control. She settled down quickly and made her brother promise he'd never sneak out of school again. Next time she'd tell her mother. Her brother never skipped school again and today he's a successful lawyer. So 20 percent self-control was enough to prevent a terrible consequence from happening. From this exercise Amber learns that she always has some self-control and her fear of losing absolutely all self-control is unfounded.

## 2. Know the Limits of Self-Control

Amber had a fear of losing control because she believed her self-control was weak. It was as if anything could push her over the edge so she had to be vigilant at all times. But what if Amber had it wrong. Is it possible that Amber's problem was not *too little self-control but too much self-control?* Could her fear of losing control be caused by trying too hard to attain unrealistic levels of control? If this is true, then reducing her self-control efforts would be the answer.

Many of Amber's experiences with fear of losing control involve unwanted, disturbing thoughts, images or impulses that pop into her mind. Amber tries hard to stop having these unwanted mental intrusions but with little success. She believes that most people don't have such horrible thoughts, and that if they do, they simply "will" them away. But what if this belief in mental control is wrong? In this case Amber is trying to reach a level of mental self-control that's impossible.

To test his out Amber could do the white bear experiment. This involves concentrating as hard as possible on thinking about a white bear for two minutes without distraction. As she's thinking hard about a white bear, she places a tick mark every time another thought pops into her mind. At the end of the two minutes, she counts up the number of tick marks which indicates how many times she was distracted from the white bear. She then repeats the exercise but this time tries hard NOT to think of a white bear for two minutes. Each time her mind wanders to the white bear she puts a tick mark. At the end of two minutes, how many times did the white bear intrude into her mind?

Amber could repeat this experiment with a variety of other thoughts and images, even the ones that upset her most, like the thought of being sexually aroused by a child. In doing the experiments, Amber discovers that she has only limited control over the thoughts and images that pop into her mind. If she asked close friends and family to do the white bear experiment, she'd come to the realization that no one has perfect self-control over their thoughts. Obviously, we have considerable control over our mind because we couldn't function if we had no control. But mental self-control is limited. It's more than 0 percent, but it's far from 100 percent. The point is we have just enough mental self-control to be productive and live in peace and harmony with others. We don't have enough mental self-control to eliminate all the thoughts that might ever trouble us and never have those thoughts again; no one does. By adopting a more realistic understanding of her self-control limits, Amber stopped pushing herself to do the impossible—to never have an unwanted intrusive thought again. The repeated failure to attain the impossible only fed her fear of losing control.

## 3. Challenge Your Self-Control

Amber avoided many situations because of her fear of losing control. This gave her opportunities to challenge her fear of losing control by doing the exact opposite of avoidance, which in CBT is called exposure. Instead of avoiding balconies, for instance, Amber worked on standing closer and closer to the handrail, even though she felt an impulse to throw herself over the railing. In the same way she forced herself to drive over suspension bridges while feeling like she might lose control of the car. And she started interacting more with the children of friends and family members despite having disgusting intrusive thoughts pop into her mind. All of these exposure experiences were powerful ways to confront her fear of losing control. Through these experiences Amber was "saying" to her fear:

*See, I do have self-control. I may feel anxious and I may have unwanted intrusive thoughts and impulses, but I am not losing control. There is nothing to fear here. I don't need to fear these intrusive thoughts and impulses because they have nothing to do with maintaining self-control. I have sufficient control of my actions to prevent undesirable consequences.*

Amber found a second set of exercises helpful in dealing with her fear of losing control. This involved taking small steps to be more spontaneous, to even dare herself to act out of character. These "dare yourself" actions seem pretty benign to most of us but for Amber they felt risky. Things like telling a joke to friends or coworkers, laughing louder and longer than normal, grimacing when a friend is talking, or butting into a conversation, to name a few actions that made her feel anxious just thinking about them. These were definitely "out of character" actions for Amber, but they taught her an important lesson. The fact that she found it so difficult to break even minor social conventions was proof that she need not fear losing control. If it was so difficult for her to be only slightly inappropriate, why fear losing control and doing something grossly inappropriate that would cause harm to herself or others? It was clear that losing control, being spontaneous and impulsive, wasn't even a part of her makeup. She couldn't lose control even when she tried in these minor interactions.

## What You Can Do

Fear of losing control isn't a factor in everyone's anxiety. If you had difficulty relating to Amber's story, then fear of losing control may not be relevant to your anxiety. Or maybe you experience times when you really do lose control of your emotions and you cause real harm to yourself or others. For you, this chapter is not relevant because your fear of losing control is realistic. This is a different type of problem that requires an entirely different therapeutic approach.

But, if like Amber, you're a very controlled person who has a deep-seated fear of losing control, then the interventions presented in this chapter are for you. As you start working on your fear, there are several issues to keep in mind.

- Catastrophic thinking is always a factor in fear of losing control. When you're anxious, you're likely jumping straight to your "nightmare scenario" of losing all control and doing something that causes significant harm or shame. To counter this, you'll need to repeatedly practice the first intervention, in which you think of degrees of control rather than a binary (*I have complete control* vs. *I have no control*).

- Of course, you can't simply talk yourself out of fear of control. The fear is too automatic, raw, and emotional. You'll also need to take action, like stop avoiding situations that trigger your fear (second intervention) and practice easing up on overcontrol (third intervention).

If you practice them with diligence and patience, the interventions in this chapter will likely help you with your fear of losing control. That said, another important contributor to fear of losing control is the experience of fear or anxiety itself. Because you are feeling anxious, you think, *There must be a real danger that I'll lose control because why else would I feel anxious?* We call this emotional reasoning and it is the subject of the next chapter.

# CHAPTER 10

# When Fear Breeds Fear

Emotional reasoning: *a bias to interpret any experience of fear, anxiety, or worry as evidence of real-life threat or danger to self or significant others.*

No doubt you've heard this phrase from the 1933 presidential inaugural address by Franklin D. Roosevelt that "we have nothing to fear except fear itself." President Roosevelt made those remarks in the context of the Great Depression, but they also have a more personal application. The reality is that most of us have a "fear bias." Not only do we find fear aversive, a feeling to avoid, but the experience of fear tends to make us even more fearful. That is, **fear tends to breed more fear.**

Have you had an experience where intense emotion takes over and causes you to imagine things that don't exist? You're in an anxiety-provoking situation, like waiting for the results of a medical test. Focusing on how anxious you feel not only makes you more anxious, but you become convinced you're about to receive bad news. As you can see from this example, emotional reasoning is more than just feeling worse by focusing on a negative emotion. The emotion feeds on itself and distorts how you interpret your experience through an unhealthy feedback loop.

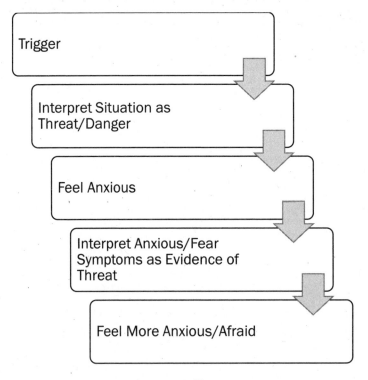

Figure 15

Once triggered by a situation that you instinctively interpret as a threat or danger to you or your loved ones, you'll naturally feel fear or anxiety. Emotional reasoning kicks in at the middle part of this feedback loop. You think, *I'm feeling anxious, so this situation must be threatening.* The fact that you feel fear or anxiety becomes the proof that the situation must be threatening. You become even more convinced that you're under threat so then the anxiety or fear intensifies. The more intense the emotion, the stronger your belief you're being threatened. In turn your anxiety increases, and the vicious cycle of emotional reasoning is set in motion.

If you've ever flown, I'm sure you can relate to this next experience of emotional reasoning. Let's say you're nervous about flying. Shortly after finding your seat, the door shuts and the flight attendant prepares the cabin for takeoff. The flight is crowded and already the air feels heavy and stifling. The plane taxis to the runway and you brace yourself for the takeoff. Your heart rate quickens, your breathing becomes more labored, you experience hot flashes and start to sweat. You're definitely feeling a rise in fear and anxiety. The takeoff is the worst and, you're convinced, the most dangerous part of flying. You brace yourself, close your eyes, say a prayer, and the plane roars down the runway. It's a smooth takeoff, and as the plane lifts you feel a slight decline in your anxiety. But shortly after takeoff the pilot cuts back on the throttle and the engines die to a whimper. You immediately think there must be a problem. Images of crashing flash through your mind and your terror accelerates. You're now in full-blown panic.

Why is the pilot's act of reducing thrust such a problem for those who feel anxious in such moments? The answer lies in emotional reasoning. If you assume that your anxiety and fear are signs of real danger, then you'll make a catastrophic interpretation, which will drive up your anxiety even further. It goes like this: *Why is the pilot cutting the engines? Something must be wrong with them. I'm terribly frightened—so I must be in a dangerous situation. If not, why would I be so afraid?* And so, fear breeds more fear. In reality, you're fine; pilots routinely cut the engines during ascension to reduce noise.

Emotional reasoning was a major contributor to the many fears and phobias that Antônia experienced. Since childhood Antônia's life has been dominated by fear. It's held her back in so many ways, greatly reduced her quality of life, and has been a large factor in her ongoing struggle with depression. To loosen the grip of fear, Antônia needed to tackle the emotional reasoning bias in her thinking. She was misreading her emotions, especially fear and anxiety. She followed her feelings without question, which led her to avoid many things because of fear.

## Antônia's Story

Fear has been a powerful emotion in Antônia's life as long as she can remember. As a child she was afraid of the dark, suffered from nightmares, and was a poor sleeper.

Now, as an adult, Antônia finds her fears more intense, causing even greater distress and interference in her life. She's become highly attuned to her emotions. Any feeling of fear or anxiety is unacceptable. She'll do anything to shut down the emotion before it gets out of hand. Nothing good comes from fear or anxiety. Antônia is a strong believer in "listen to your heart" with feelings being the most reliable guide of the heart. So, when feelings of anxiety or fear arise, Antônia believes she must take them seriously; that they are telling her harm or danger was just ahead unless she takes preventive action.

This way of thinking about her emotions provided fertile soil for emotional reasoning. Her biased thinking about emotions, but especially fear, had a negative impact on her quality of life and happiness. Antônia can't fly because of her anxiety. The last time she attempted a flight she had a full-blown panic attack and swore she'd never fly again. Despite what she heard about flying being the safest mode of transportation, the intensity of her fear told her otherwise. Her "heart" was telling her, *Antônia stay on the ground; the next time you fly you could crash.*

Antônia was also a nervous driver. Again, she interpreted her anxiety as evidence that driving was a dangerous activity. This caused her to overcompensate, which had a negative effect on her driving skills. For example, she was so afraid of being rear-ended that she constantly looked in her rearview mirror. Once in heavy, stop-and-start traffic, she rear-ended the car in front of her because she was staring at the car quickly approaching from behind. In another example of emotional reasoning, Antônia avoided crowded malls or stores because they made her uncomfortable. She took this anxiety as a sign of real possibility that public places had become unsafe. Once again, she concluded, *Better to avoid than put yourself in harm's way.*

## Corrective Strategies

Recently, Antônia sought therapy for the first time. Her therapist recommended a few strategies to help her deal with the emotional reasoning bias at the heart of her fear, anxiety, and avoidance. These included practicing an attentional shift strategy to reduce her intense focus on feelings, conducting an investigation to determine whether the anxiety is a true or false signal of impending danger, and taking a course of action that challenges the emotional reasoning bias.

### 1. Attentional Shift

The first step in countering the emotional reasoning bias is to focus your attention on what's happening around you. When Antônia felt anxious or fearful, she became totally focused on her feelings. Whatever was happening around her faded from view as she became totally immersed in the emotion. It's easy to get caught in emotional reasoning when your attention becomes so narrowly focused. To break out of this myopic mindset, Antônia had to learn to broaden her perspective to include what was happening around her. By doing this she could reframe or understand her fear within the context of her present environment. There is a two-step process to this form of attentional shifting:

   a.  Acknowledge what you are feeling within the present context. Say to yourself, *I am feeling* (afraid, anxious, frustrated) *while* (state here your current activity). For her part, Antônia would often acknowledge the feelings she was experiencing as they arose, but she would stop there. By also including the context, the current activity, you are making the feeling specific to the situation.

b.   Shift your attention to the context. Describe what is happening around you, the physical characteristics of your environment, the people around you, the input from your five senses (see, hear, smell, touch, taste). Be as specific and detailed as possible. If your attention shifts back to the fear, acknowledge the fear, but then return to doing a mental accounting of your environment.

Antônia could use this strategy when going to a crowded supermarket after work. This is the mental account she might make of her surroundings.

*I'm feeling anxious entering this supermarket. It is more crowded than I expected. I can feel my heart beating faster, I feel lightheaded, tense, and fidgety, and I want to run. But I'm just standing here in the supermarket, reaching for a shopping cart (acknowledged the feeling in the present context). I grip the handle of the cart and start to push it. Oh great, one of the wheels is dragging. I start down the produce aisle. I notice the cool air in the store and I already feel like I can breathe better compared to the hot, sticky air when walking from the parking lot. I'm looking over the fruit, making sure what I select is fresh. I pick through the fruit and feel the texture of each, taking particular notice of their ripeness. As I continue shopping, I look carefully for the expiration date of each item before placing it in the shopping cart. I take particular notice of the other customers in the store, what they wear, their facial expressions, and what they put in their shopping carts (attentional shift to present context). My attention shifts back to my anxiety. The lightheadedness is gone, I'm a little less tense and my breathing is regular. Okay, let's get back to what I'd doing and where I am. Pay attention to my surroundings. I don't want to run into anyone with my cart.*

As Antônia practiced shifting her attention from her fear/anxiety to her surroundings, she was subtly invalidating her fear. There was definitely some stress associated with a crowded supermarket, but was there really any danger that justified her fear?

## 2. Investigate and Evaluate

While paying attention to your environment, make a mental note of anything that looks threatening, suspicious, or upsetting. Alternatively, what do you see in your environment that indicates it's safe? As Antônia proceeded down the aisles of the supermarket, there were several things that made her feel uncomfortable. There was a group of teenagers who seemed loud and rather belligerent. A large middle-aged man looked angry and upset; some people were rushing about and not careful with their shopping carts. And then there was a long line at the checkout and Antônia had too many items for the self-serve checkout. As she thought more deeply about all of these factors, she realized they made her feel uncomfortable but they were not indicators of some threat to her physical safety.

She then forced herself to look for signs of safety. In reality no one even noticed her; they were all too busy, absorbed in their grocery shopping. The security guard in the store was just wandering around. He clearly didn't think there was anyone suspicious in the store. All the staff were focused on their work. No one looked worried or fearful. And there were several elderly ladies doing their shopping. They did not look the least bit scared. As she summed up the evidence of "imagined threat" vs. safety, Antônia concluded the assumption of safety was a better match to the circumstance than the assumption of danger.

Could the situation change instantly? Absolutely! But at the moment, safety was a more accurate assumption than threat. Her anxiety and fear in the supermarket were a false alarm.

## 3. False Alarms

Fear is necessary for our survival; it signals danger, warning us to take preventive action. If you're driving in the winter and suddenly lose control of the car, you instantly feel fear. You regain control of the car, but the fear lingers. You then test the road to see if it's full of black ice. In this scenario, fear is a useful and valid emotion. It may cause you to slow down or even cut short your trip because of hazardous road conditions it'd be better not to risk.

Unfortunately, fear and anxiety often give false warnings. You may feel anxious about driving even though there's hardly any traffic and the road conditions are excellent. So how do you know when your fear is genuine, signaling a real-life threat, and when it's a false alarm?

One way to tell true from false warnings is to look for the origins or cause of the fear or anxiety. We all do this instinctively when we're fearful or anxious, but you can't rely on that first automatic response if the fear system in your brain gives off lots of false warnings. Instead, you have to take a hard, thoughtful second look at the possible origins of your fear, anxiety or worry. This is what Antônia needed to do every time she felt anxious because she knew her brain was generating lots of false warnings. When she felt a surge of fear or anxiety, she asked herself the following questions:

a.  Is this a situation that would make most people feel anxious, fearful, or worried?

b.  If I avoid this situation, am I significantly reducing my risk of harm, injury, or death?

c.  If I listen to my fear or anxiety and avoid/leave this situation, is my quality of life and independence negatively affected?

d.  If I remain in this situation and ignore my fear/anxiety, will it make me stronger and more resilient? Is the fear/anxiety likely to eventually fade on its own? Like a false burglar alarm, will my brain learn to reset its sensitivity, so it becomes more accurate?

When Antônia asked herself these questions when she became anxious in the supermarket, she answered **no** to questions (a) and (b) and **yes** to questions (c) and (d). Clearly her anxiety in the supermarket was a false warning. Like a false burglar alarm, the best response was to ignore the anxiety and get on with her shopping.

## 4. Plan of Action

Let's say you've decided that your fear or anxiety in a situation is false; that it arises from within you and not some real-life danger. You realize that leaving the situation, giving in to the fear or anxiety, only makes it stronger and reinforces your emotional reasoning bias. After deciding that your fear is a false alarm, the next step is to plan out a course of action that is consistent with a false alarm approach. This involves taking a detached observer perspective, letting your fear or anxiety ebb and flow naturally while continuing with an activity in the present moment. By letting the fear, anxiety, or worry fade on its own, you're overriding the emotional reasoning bias. You're like the police officer ignoring a burglar alarm that you know is the result of a faulty alarm system. There is no burglary in progress, so why bother with it?

Antônia used this strategy to deal with her anxiety about driving. Of course, accidents do happen and sometimes they are fatal, but she also knew that she could not trust her anxiety to alert her to real dangers on the road. Her fear system was misfiring at a high rate, giving her a steady stream of false signals. So she decided to change her driving habits so she was not giving in to her fear. She worked on spending more time looking ahead rather than in the rearview mirror. She increased her speed so she was driving closer to the speed limit and she practiced passing slow-moving vehicles using the passing lane. She also volunteered to drive when going places with friends, and she did not avoid congested traffic when doing errands. In this way Antônia's actions were in direct contradiction with her emotional reasoning bias. Instead of "fear breeding more fear," her actions weakened the hold of fear on her life.

# What You Can Do

Maybe this chapter is an eye-opener for you. You've been working on your anxiety but never realized that the emotional reasoning bias was part of the problem. You've been treating each experience of fear and anxiety as if it always signalled harm or danger. When you treat fear and anxiety that signals a false threat like it was real, it will only make these feelings more intense. The possibility that your fear system is generating false signals is a new way of thinking about your emotions.

You can't overcome the emotional reasoning bias until you're convinced that much of your fear, anxiety, or worry is a false alarm. If you think every experience of anxiety is an accurate reflection of reality, you won't bother trying to figure out if the experience is a true or false alarm. You'll just slip into the emotional reasoning bias (*if I'm afraid, I must be in danger*). One way to work on changing your attitude about fear and anxiety is to keep track of your experiences and their outcome. After several weeks, look back on what you wrote. How often did you feel afraid or anxious in situations that reflected a high possibility of harm (true alarm) and how often did you have fear/anxiety in situations but nothing bad happened even when you stayed in the situation (false alarm)? Through this exercise you'll learn whether "false alarm fear/anxiety" is a problem fostering an emotional reasoning bias. Once this is determined, you can use the strategies discussed in this chapter to ensure that fear does not breed fear.

The emotional reasoning bias is like a silent intruder. It can affect your anxiety level without your being aware of its impact. In the next chapter we consider a process that is much more obvious. It's an unhealthy way of coping with anxiety that makes little sense except to those who believe in its power. It's called *neutralization* and it's based on the influence of ritual and repetition over our emotions.

# CHAPTER 11

# Old Habits Die Hard

*Neutralization: a conscious, effortful, and habitual way of thinking or acting that serves to reduce the likelihood of some anticipated negative experience that causes you to feel anxious or worried.*

Do you have unhealthy habits, like eating sugary treats, drinking too much coffee, smoking or vaping, or spending too much time on social media? You're aware of their negative effects and you've tried to cut back but your will power collapses. You can't seem to help yourself. Did you know that unhealthy habits can also play a role in anxiety? When you're living an anxious life, it's easy to rely on one or two coping responses that seem to relieve the anxiety, at least in the short term. If you use these coping responses repeatedly, they can take on a ritualistic form, which in the end only make your anxiety problem worse.

How often have you left your house or apartment and had the thought, *Did I lock the door?* Maybe you immediately put your mind at ease by thinking, *Of course I locked the door. I always lock the door when I leave. It's a well-learned habit.* But what happens if that reassuring thought fails, and you continue to doubt that you locked the door. Now your anxiety builds because you think, *If it's unlocked, someone could break in and steal my stuff.* This perceived threat, along with the doubt, causes a further rise in your anxiety. So, what do you do? The logical thing is to go back and check. You check the door and discover it's locked. Immediately your anxiety drops, and you leave.

Checking is a form of neutralization because it brings relief from your anxiety. There are many ways you can neutralize anxiety, such as redoing an action to ensure you did it right, rereading text several times to make sure you understand it, rearranging stuff so it's in the right order, thinking a positive thought to cancel the effects of a negative thought, reciting a prayer, repeating a reassuring phrase, and the like. Although these responses seem quite different, they all share the same function: to reduce or eliminate anxious feelings. When you check, for instance, you might think, *There, the door is locked; someone is less likely to break in and steal my stuff.* For some people with obsessive-compulsive disorder (OCD), one check does not reduce their anxiety or doubt, and so they go back again and again to check if the door is locked. Now checking becomes a problem in its own right and it feeds into your anxiety about unlocked doors.

Is there something you do **repeatedly** in an effort to feel less anxious? If so, it's probably a neutralization ritual.

Every neutralization ritual is built on a false belief. Let's take a look at our "locked door" example. To repeatedly check the door, you'd have to believe that you can't trust yourself, that you have a habit of leaving doors unlocked. But is that true? Do you tend to walk away and leave your door unlocked? Or is this a false belief? You could test out this belief by doing a random, infrequent test. It would involve going back to check if the door is locked whether you have doubts or not. (Only do this a few times. You don't want to create a checking compulsion.) How neutralization makes anxiety worse depends on the interaction of several processes.

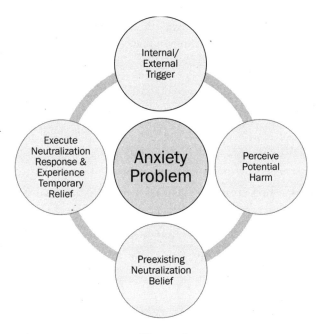

Figure 16

The processes illustrated in this figure are relevant to problematic anxiety. This is anxiety that is unusually intense, persistent, and disproportionate to the situation in which it occurs. In our current discussion, neutralization rituals cause an increase in the intensity and persistence of anxiety through four processes. First, there is a trigger that sets everything in motion. This could be an external situation, like touching something you think is dirty like a doorknob to a public washroom, or an internal thought, image, or impulse like thinking your email might be taken the wrong way by the receiver. The trigger is instantly interpreted as causing potential harm or injury. In the case of touching a doorknob, the harm perception would be fear of contamination; with the work email, the perception is that of bad relations between you and the person receiving the email. Once there is an interpretation of potential harm, anxiety rises.

For people who neutralize when feeling anxious, anxiety immediately activates beliefs in the power of neutralization. After touching a "contaminated doorknob," you might wash your hands repeatedly to get rid of possible germs on your hands. For the email you might go back and reread your email several times to reassure yourself that the message could not be interpreted wrongly. In these examples, washing and rereading are neutralization rituals. The execution of these rituals causes a temporary reduction in anxiety. Unfortunately, this relief also reinforces your belief that the triggers are potentially harmful and so the entire cycle is set to repeat itself. Over time, your anxiety problem builds as other processes like reassurance seeking and avoidance contribute to making anxiety worse.

The insidious effects of neutralization can be seen in Martin's anxiety-driven OCD. He had an intense fear of contamination and got hopelessly stuck in washing compulsions that made daily living intolerable. To break free of his OCD, Martin needed to change his false beliefs about the washing compulsions and use preventive strategies to wean himself off cleaning rituals. He knew the handwashing was excessive, but he was powerless to "just say no."

## Martin's Story

Martin called himself a "germaphobe." He talked about having an intense fear of germs that started while in his late teens. Now in his mid-thirties Martin's fear of contamination and relentless urge to wash and clean are causing havoc in his life. Several years ago, Martin was diagnosed with OCD. His type of OCD is especially relevant for understanding anxiety because his compulsions are driven by a desire to reduce the intense anxiety felt when he worries about possible exposure to germs. To deal with his anxiety, Martin washes his hands repeatedly, takes long showers, launders his clothes several times a day, and wipes objects down with alcohol. All of these actions are neutralization responses because they're intended to lower his anxiety about possible contamination.

It's easy to see how Martin fell into the neutralization trap. Think for a moment what happens when your hands are dirty, feel sticky, or you wonder if you came into contact with something that could be germy. The natural response is to give your hands a thorough wash. If you're thinking the object you touched might have germs that could cause sickness, you might also use a hand sanitizer. But Martin's anxiety-driven OCD went far beyond the normal. Practically everything outside his home triggered his contamination fear, and one wash was never enough. In fact, his handwashing got so frequent and intense that his hands often bled and blistered. His compulsions or neutralization became so intense that he'd spend hours each day cleaning, washing, and wiping down any object he thought might be contaminated.

By the time Martin sought therapy, practically anything outside his home was a potential contaminant. He had a false belief that germs would increase his risk of cancer. His OCD became much worse during the COVID-19 pandemic. He now had proof that public places and any association with people posed extreme danger of contagion. The virus was everywhere, and Martin went to great lengths to protect himself and his partner. He kept their household well-stocked with personal protective equipment (PPE), and he would constantly use alcohol to wipe down anything his partner touched because he had come home after interacting with the public. Gradually, Martin became housebound, unable to work or even keep a doctor's appointment when he did become ill. He depended on his partner for everything to do with the outside world, which of course put an enormous strain on their relationship.

The number of situations that trigger Martin's fear is endless. Some examples include garbage cans, the landline telephone, dirty dishes in the dishwasher, any exterior doorknob, retrieving food from the refrigerator, touching delivery parcels, driving in the car, close proximity to strangers, and the like. Each of these situations elicit intense fear and Martin's reaction is to neutralize: to wash, shower, or clean objects with alcohol wipes. The compulsion continues until Martin feels less anxious. This indicates "the danger" is averted, but within a few minutes something else reignites his fear and the cycle starts all over. For example, he takes a carton of milk from the refrigerator. Immediately he thinks, *That milk came from the store. Lots of people handled that carton. Did I really get rid of all the germs? Maybe it still has germs and now I've touched it.* This thought process causes intense anxiety, which then sets in motion Martin's washing and cleaning compulsions. In this way the neutralization compulsions maintain Martin's intense fear of contamination.

## Prevention Strategies

Neutralization responses are difficult to break because they become automatic responses aimed at relieving anxiety. It's an unhealthy habit you might think could be broken with an extra dose of willpower. But it takes more than willpower to stop neutralizing. You also need to employ strategies that work, like a graduated, systematic program of response prevention, delay tactics, and helpful beliefs about neutralization.

### 1. The Difficulty Ladder

You were introduced to fear exposure in chapter 3. If you recall, Jamal first created a hierarchy of fear situations that he avoided. Martin also created a fear exposure hierarchy using the same strategy to tackle his neutralization rituals, but with an important difference. (See http://www.newharbinger.com/53165 for the worksheet.) Like Jamal, he started by listing twenty or so situations that made him feel anxious. Most of these situations he would avoid but when exposed to them he always engaged in a washing or cleaning compulsion. Because neutralization prevention was the goal of Martin's intervention, he arranged these situations in ascending order according to the strength of his neutralization urge. A 0–10 scale was used where 0 = "no urge to neutralize" (engage in washing compulsion), 5 = "moderately strong urge," to 10 = "irresistible urge to neutralize." The urge to wash was based on Martin's belief that the situation posed possible harm (*Did I come in contact with germs that could make me seriously ill?*) and that washing would eliminate the potential harm and relieve his anxiety. So Martin created a "difficulty ladder" where the urge to neutralize would be more intense with situations higher in the hierarchy. The following is a sample of Martin's neutralization hierarchy.

| Triggers | Intensity of Neutralization Urge |
|---|---|
| Sitting in a crowded doctor's office | 10 |
| Eating food in a mall food court | 9 |
| Opening doors in public places with bare hands | 9 |
| Eating in an upscale restaurant | 8 |
| Using gas pumps with bare hands | 6 |
| Touching my own garbage cans barehanded on collection day | 6 |
| Picking up delivered packages with bare hands | 5 |
| Putting dirty dishes in dishwasher | 3 |
| Touching newly purchased food packages | 2 |
| Touching cupboard doorknobs | 1 |

Martin's difficulty ladder guided the rest of his treatment. Starting at the very bottom of the ladder would be a waste of time because Martin could stop the washing rituals in these situations if he just put a little effort into it. Instead, he started with situations higher up on the ladder such as putting dirty dishes in the dishwasher or picking up delivery parcels with his bare hands. His neutralization urge was quite strong in these situations, so he needed to use various strategies to stop the cleaning rituals. Let's take picking up delivered parcels with bare hands as our example.

## 2. Cold Turkey vs. Tapering

Martin knew that his fear of germs was excessive and completely out of touch with reality. Everyone touches doorknobs, for example, and they don't become seriously ill—at least, not from touching doorknobs. Also, Martin knew that washing his hands repeatedly was no guarantee that all germs were eliminated. He didn't use a scanner or powder to detect germs because he had a feeling this would drive him further into his OCD. Instead, he washed until he felt some relief; that was a noticeable drop in anxiety.

Martin also knew that to stop compulsive washing "cold turkey" was not reasonable. He had tried this numerous times and always failed. Friends and family would tell him to "just stop washing," but they failed to appreciate the intensity of his urge to wash. As an alternative, he adopted a "tapering approach." As he moved up the difficulty ladder, with each situation, Martin would also taper his withdrawal from washing and cleaning. This was how it worked with the parcel delivery situation. Martin's goal was to handle parcels with bare hands without subsequent washing, use of hand sanitizers, or alcohol wipes. He decided that stopping hand washing would be hardest, so he first cut out hand sanitizers and alcohol wipes. For two weeks (delivery parcels arrived almost daily), he continued to wash his hands after handling parcels but refrained from hand sanitizers or alcohol wipes. Next, he worked on a gradual delay in washing his hands after handling a parcel. Instead of immediately washing his hands, he delayed it by five minutes. Once he felt confident in tolerating the urge to wash for five minutes, he increased the delay to ten minutes. He continued in this manner over several weeks until the delay was great enough that the urge to wash and its associated anxiety had declined. Granted, often some other potential contaminant happened in the meantime that diverted Martin's attention away from the parcel handling. But the fact that he was able to tolerate the urge to wash that had once been immediate and overwhelming was meaningful on its own.

Of course, one of the disadvantages of tapering your prevention efforts is that treatment progress is slow. It can take many months as you learn to tolerate the urge to neutralize for one fear situation after another. It took Martin months to work through all the situations in his "difficulty ladder." But tapering has many advantages as well. You are more likely to succeed in eliminating your neutralization rituals. You're less likely to become overwhelmed with anxiety and neutralization urges and give up on yourself. Tapering is also more flexible, so you can go back and taper a little less aggressively if the current level is too difficult.

## 3. Boosting Motivation

Despite the many advantages of tapering, it takes considerable courage to face your fears and stop relying on neutralization to relieve anxiety. You'll need to believe in the importance of neutralization prevention to stick with your program. To maintain a high level of motivation, a deeper understanding of the powerful effects of neutralization rituals is required.

Have you ever tried to cut down on eating certain foods that aren't so good for you? Most of us have at one time or another. Do you find it easier to resist the craving for this food the more you give into it? Probably just the opposite. The more you give in to the craving and eat the food you're trying not to eat, the more of it you eat. The same with using neutralization rituals to relieve anxiety. The more you do it, the tighter the connection between anxiety and neutralization.

Martin was able to see this connection in the ups and downs of his OCD. When he was on medication, the urge to wash was less intense so he washed less. At the same time his anxiety decreased. Unfortunately, his avoidance didn't change as much, so he was still avoiding many of the things that triggered his fear of germs. Nevertheless, he was able to see that whenever his neutralization rituals (washing and cleaning) declined, so did the anxiety and vice versa. This indicated that neutralization prevention would have a positive impact on his anxiety and fear.

Martin became more convinced of the importance of neutralization prevention after doing a little experiment. While tapering his handwashing after handling a parcel, he rated his anxiety at fifteen-minute intervals for two hours. At the same time, he did the same fifteen-minute ratings after touching the trash container in the kitchen. Here he did not delay handwashing. He kept these ratings over a two-week period and then compared the results. What Martin discovered is that after two weeks, his anxiety when touching the parcels was significantly lower than the anxiety he felt after touching the trash container. He also made another surprising discovery. Often handwashing after touching the trash container did not relieve his anxiety quickly. Sometimes his anxiety persisted or even increased because he was unsure if his handwashing was adequate. So he would get caught into repeated handwashing until he felt some relief. This little experiment convinced Martin of the importance of reducing handwashing in treating his anxiety-driven OCD.

## 4. Delay Tactics

Chapter 3 discussed various strategies useful in coping with high levels of anxiety. These same strategies can be used to tolerate the anxiety you'll feel when you delay or completely eliminate your neutralizing ritual. Martin found distraction especially helpful in sticking to his tapering program. After touching something that aroused his fear of contamination, Martin resisted handwashing but, as expected, his anxiety rose. In such moments, he would distract himself by engaging in a physical activity that required considerable attention. For example, he washed the car, tidied up the garage, initiated a house repair, and the like. While doing these activities, his anxiety remained elevated, but it was more tolerable than if he sat in a chair and tried to resist the urge to wash. If while doing the distracting activity, Martin became aware of his anxiety, he practiced mindful acceptance of his anxious thoughts and feelings (see chapter 3 for details).

# What You Can Do

Most of the elements of anxiety are relatively easy to identify. Avoidance, catastrophizing, and reassurance seeking, for example, are quite obvious. But neutralizing is different. Still, if you engage in compulsive rituals when anxious (like repeated washing, checking, or redoing) your neutralization might be straightforward. Using compulsion-prevention strategies will be an important ingredient in your therapy.

Neutralization can also be more subtle and more difficult to identify. Examples of subtle neutralizing include (a) repeating certain words, phrases, or prayers when anxious, (b) replacing an anxious thought with a special positive thought, (c) analyzing the meaning of an anxious thought, (d) endlessly reassuring yourself you'll be alright, (e) being self-critical for feeling anxious, (f) engaging in thought stopping or suppression, or (g) imagining a comfortable or safe place. Some of these responses look healthy, but they actually contribute to anxiety when they become ritualistic.

If you're unsure if your way of coping with anxiety has become an unhealthy neutralization response, ask yourself the following questions:

- Do I have certain coping responses to anxiety that I use repeatedly? Has it become a type of ritual for dealing with anxiety?

- Do I feel compelled (an urge) to use this coping response when anxious? Do I feel I have to execute the response when anxious and it has to be done in a certain way?

- If I don't engage in the coping response, does the anxiety become intolerable?

- Do I feel some relief after engaging in the coping ritual?

If you answered "yes" to most of these questions, consider working on your neutralization rituals as part of your anxiety reduction therapy by creating a difficulty hierarchy and then gradually delaying the neutralization.

Before concluding our discussion of the basic elements of anxiety and its treatment, the final chapter considers one more unhealthy coping strategy that makes anxiety worse rather than better.

# CHAPTER 12

# Can't Let Go

Post-Event Processing: *repeated and irresistible reanalysis of a past social experience to obtain anxiety-relieving self-reassurance that you did not say or do something that you might now regret.*

Have you ever worried "obsessively" that you might have said something in a social setting that is embarrassing, or even shameful? Maybe for days or even weeks after the event you keep rehashing over and over in your mind whether you said something that you now regret. Your anxiety and worry rise whenever you think about the experience because you can't be certain whether your words or actions were inappropriate or not. If you did say something that was inappropriate or hurtful toward another person, you might feel a variety of negative emotions like anxiety, guilt, regret, embarrassment, or shame. This experience of "obsessive" thinking of a past anxiety-provoking event is called post-event processing.

The term "post-event" refers to a type of fretting done after a social experience. It's called "processing" because you're "obsessively" trying to recall every detail of an interaction, what you said and how others responded to determine whether your actions or words were okay or not. The problem is that memory is not perfect and so you keep going over the event repeatedly in your mind, looking for new clues that would relieve your doubts. But post-event processing usually has the opposite effect. Instead of relieving doubt and feeling better, you feel more anxious because you can never attain the level of certainty that what you said or did was appropriate. Maybe someone was offended by your remarks, or maybe they're highly critical, concluding that you must be ignorant, rude, unstable, or stupid. You can't be sure, so you keep trying to recall details of the experience, but the more you do this, the more anxious and worried you feel.

Take the following example. You're at a work-related social event. You hate chit-chatting and you try to avoid these informal social events, but this is the year-end holiday party and you must make an appearance. You feel self-conscious, awkward, and anxious, so you drink a little more than usual. You're in a small group of coworkers and the conversation gets quite lively around office politics. Normally, you would say little and guard your words carefully. But on this occasion, your tongue loosens and you disclose a couple of incidents involving your manager that make him look incompetent and foolish. Everyone laughs and this starts a cascade of other stories in which the manager becomes a laughingstock. You don't think anything of this whole incident until the next morning. As you think back to the social event, a sick feeling builds in your stomach and you can feel the anxiety mount. *What exactly did I say about my manager? Did I betray a secret or at least an incident that should have been kept private? What if it gets back to the manager that I was making fun of him? What do my coworkers now think of me? Do they think I'm mean, insensitive, someone who can't be trusted? Of course, everyone was laughing and telling stories, but I started it. Does that make me the ringleader?* You start ruminating about last night, searching your memory to answer these questions. But most of these questions have no answer, and they certainly can't be addressed by recalling some hidden memory. Thus, your anxiety builds the longer you try to satisfy your doubts and concerns. Here's how post-event processing increases anxiety and worry.

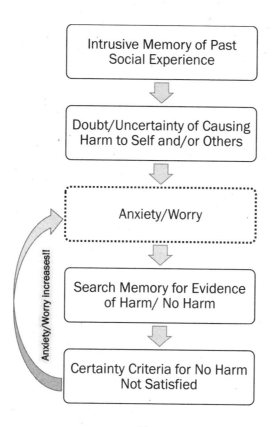

Figure 17

Post-event processing starts with a memory or recollection of a previous social experience that pops into your mind. This gives rise to doubt, uncertainty over what you said or did that might have caused harm to you or to others. For example, you might question whether you were an embarrassment. Did you bring shame or humiliation upon yourself? Did you say or do something that you later regret or that could have a negative consequence? Will others criticize you or think less of you because of your remarks? All of this is a type of harm to self. There's also harm to others, which involves uncertainty over whether you said something rude, offensive, or inappropriate to others that reflects badly on you. The doubt or uncertainty about harm triggers anxiety or worry. To relieve this initial bout of anxiety, you search your memory for clues that no harm was done to yourself or others. This memory search is the core element of post-event processing. It could last just a few minutes or many hours or even days or weeks. But the harder you try to recall something that indicates "all is well," the less likely you'll find evidence that makes you feel certain you caused no harm. The memory rehearsal becomes a vicious cycle that feeds back into your anxiety and worry, making the whole experience more intense and enduring. Rather than squelching your anxiety and worry, it fuels your distress.

## Hana's Story

Hana has felt anxious in social situations for as long as she can remember. She's always been on the shy side and developed a fear of bringing shame on herself and others. Raised in a family where respect, integrity, and deference were emphasized, Hana developed a keen sense of sensitivity to others and her effect on their emotional state. She decided early in life that it was best to be quiet and not make waves. She typically dislikes the attention of others, preferring instead to fade into the background.

As a child Hana was shy and self-conscious around her peers and found it exceedingly difficult to make friends. School was a highly anxiety-provoking experience but she got through it.

Hana now works as a corporate lawyer for a large insurance company. But social anxiety remains a perennial problem. She tries to keep to herself but of course it's impossible to avoid all social interaction, especially at work. So when she does speak, she'll often spend days after going over in her mind what she said that might have offended others. The more she reflects on her past conversations, the more anxious and worried she feels about offending others. Her main fear is that she will say something rude or offensive to others. Her finely tuned sensitivity to the needs of others causes her to be hypervigilant to the reactions of people during social interactions. For Hana the ultimate disaster is being responsible for causing others to feel shame or humiliation. Of course, the legal profession is inherently adversarial, so Hana is always second-guessing herself, wondering if she's pushed too far and shamed her adversary.

Post-event processing is the main coping strategy Hana uses to deal with her social anxiety. She can spend hours rehashing in her mind the details of past interactions: *Did I come across too strong? Was I too critical? Did they take it personally? Was there any indication they were upset with me? Did I cause the person to feel embarrassed or ashamed? I can't be a good person if I'm causing pain and suffering to other people.*

Of course, the hours spent reliving past social interactions did not relieve Hana's anxiety. Instead, she felt more upset and anxious because proof that she was not offensive was elusive. She could never be convinced she didn't offend because she couldn't get into the mind of other people. Post-event processing came naturally to Hana given her highly analytical mind. But it was also her greatest downfall. To overcome her social anxiety, she needed to stop rehashing the past. Fortunately for Hana, there are several strategies she can use to reduce her dependency on post-event processing.

## How to Stop Spinning

There are several ways that Hana can build a program to stop overanalyzing past social interactions. They include (a) reexamining her history of offending others to determine the likelihood that she is an "offensive person," (b) decatastrophizing the consequences of being rude, insensitive, or offensive,

(c) listing the immediate and long-term costs of embarrassment, and (d) generating an alternative, more realistic narrative of a past social experience.

## 1. Take a History

Anxiety is about threat, whether real or imagined. So Hana's work on post-event processing had to start at the beginning; was her fear of offending people realistic, imagined, or exaggerated? If she's a rude and insensitive person who is often offensive to others—and there are people like this—then she'll need to work on personality issues and her interpersonal style. But if her fear of offending others is based on an imagined possibility that she is offensive, this is a very different problem. No amount of post-event analysis will address this imagined fear.

To settle the question of real vs. imagined fear, Hana listed all social experiences where she recalled feeling anxious and then getting stuck in post-event processing. (See http://www.newharbinger.com/53165 for the worksheet.) These could be recent experiences as well as past events that stretched back to her childhood. The following are some of the social experiences Hana listed.

- Disclosed details about private interactions with manager that made coworkers at party laugh.

- Clicked dislike on a friend's posting on social media.

- In middle school, joined with other classmates in laughing at a girl's poor presentation. The girl looked hurt and upset by the experience.

- Teased by older sister and replied that she was fat and ugly.

- Recently wrote a legal opinion that was highly critical of a colleague's compliance report.

Beside each experience Hana was asked to write down "hard evidence" that she offended the other person. Hard evidence included anything said or a change in behavior or facial expression that indicated she offended the person. Feelings or worries of offense didn't count. As an example, let's take the last experience that Hana listed. Nothing was ever said by her colleague that he was offended by her critique of his compliance brief. It was normal practice for the legal team to critique each other's work. In fact, thinking more closely, Hana recalled that her colleague had later thanked her for pointing out some serious shortcomings in his brief. Several days later they had coffee together and all seemed well between them. There was no "hard evidence" he was offended or felt shamed by her critique.

As Hana went through each social experience looking for hard evidence that she offended people, more times than not she came up empty-handed. On the one or two occasions where there was some evidence that the person was troubled by what Hana said, there was no evidence the distress was significant or long-lasting. Clearly Hana's problem was more imagined than realistic.

This exercise helped Hana realize that post-event processing could not be helpful in relieving her social anxiety. So much of what came up in her processing was distorted—more her feelings or mistaken impressions of a moment than reality. From that point, whenever Hana started to ruminate on past events, she could remind herself of the exercise: *I'm not the type of person who goes around offending people; this fear is more likely imagined than real.*

## 2. Count the Cost

Social anxiety can stem from a variety of fears. For some, like Hana, it is a fear of upsetting others. But there are other fears that can drive social anxiety, like fear of (a) feeling embarrassed, shamed, or humiliated; (b) being criticized; or (c) experiencing the disapproval or rejection of others. What's common in each case is a belief that the consequences of the feared state are severe, maybe even life-changing. But is this really true? Take your worst social experience of shame, criticism, disapproval, or offense. How has this experience changed your life? Has it really been a costly experience? Important: When doing this exercise, exclude your interactions with partners and family members. Romantic and family experiences can be life-changing because of the unique roles partners and family members play in our lives. Social anxiety, on the other hand, is usually *outside* our closest relationships, so these are the experiences relevant to post-event processing.

For Hana the worst experience of possible offense happened a couple of years ago. Her legal team was meeting with senior management, and one of her colleagues made a presentation detailing a negotiation strategy the corporation should take in an acquisition bid. During the Q & A period, Hana raised a fundamental flaw in her colleague's strategy. It was an omission that the colleague should have noticed. She was clearly upset and embarrassed by the mistake. Hana could feel the pain and embarrassment her colleague felt in front of management. It was a very uncomfortable moment for everyone.

What were the immediate and long-term consequences of this incident for Hana? Again she was asked to list the realistic, the actual consequences of the event, not how it felt. What were the personal costs for raising this issue with her colleague's presentation? Were the consequences significant, enduring, and intolerable? Here's what she listed.

- For two weeks Suzanne (the colleague) would not speak to me. She seemed to avoid me at every opportunity.

- Since that day whenever I make presentations, Suzanne always has something negative to say. It used to be worse than it is now, though.

- It's taken time but Suzanne is no longer hostile toward me. We are cordial to each other and have been able to work together on projects, though she is cool toward me.

- I'm now asked by senior management to review all acquisition contracts.

- Other corporate lawyers ask for my opinion on their work.

- There's been no change in how my team treats me.

- I still get excellent performance reviews and year-end bonuses.

After reviewing the realistic outcome associated with her "worst incident of offense," Hana realized she greatly exaggerates the significance and long-term impact of an offense. People may be momentarily upset, but over time it fades in significance. They have more important challenges in their life than whether or not they were offended by what you said. So when Hana started to engage in post-event processing, she reminded herself that what's important to her is not necessarily important to someone else. She mindfully reflected on the following realization.

*Rehashing the past will settle nothing and only make me more anxious. I'll never be able to convince myself whether I was offensive or not. Going over and over the details only causes me to catastrophize the possible offense. It's best to assume that if I did offend someone, it's no big deal to them. And if it is a big deal, they'll be sure to let me know either directly or through someone else.*

## 3. Confront Fear of Embarrassment

Embarrassment is one of the most distressing emotions we experience. Most of us will do almost anything to avoid embarrassment. But people differ in how much they fear embarrassment. Some are so frightened they avoid drawing any attention to themselves because they might blush and that would be embarrassing. At the other extreme are people who seem impervious to embarrassment. We call them shameless. Hana had a strong fear of embarrassment and it made her shy and anxious around others. It also contributed to post-event processing because she reanalyzed past experiences to determine if she said or did something embarrassing.

Like most people with social anxiety, Hana exaggerated the consequences of an embarrassing experience. As a result she believed it was important to determine whether or not she did something embarrassing.

Her modus operandi for settling this question was post-event processing. But like all the other fears, this strategy can never truly settle the question. To stop this unhealthy coping strategy, Hana had to learn to accept that embarrassment was always a possibility but its effects were momentary at best.

Once again Hana used the CBT strategy of decatastrophizing to confront her fear of embarrassment. It starts by writing down a recent embarrassing experience. For Hana it was being late for an important meeting. The meeting started and Hana had to walk in and sit near the front. The presenter stopped talking and everyone looked at her. Hana felt her face turning bright red, a rush of hot flashes coursed through her body, and her anxiety spiked. She was sure everyone noticed her flustered state. Next Hana took a hard look at the consequences of her embarrassment. As uncomfortable as she felt in the moment, was it really that significant? She questioned the experience by asking:

- My colleagues noticed I was embarrassed, but is there any evidence this has changed their opinion of me? Do they really think less of me because I had an embarrassing moment?

- Has my life changed in any meaningful way because of the embarrassment? Is it really a significant defining moment like losing my job, being diagnosed with a serious medical illness, or breakup of an intimate relationship?

- Has walking in late to the meeting caused my work colleagues to permanently think less of me? Will they really think, "Hana is such a competent, helpful, and respectful person, but I can't believe she was late to that meeting and looked embarrassed. Clearly, she's an emotionally fragile person. I've changed my opinion of her"?

- Has my opinion of someone changed because they had an embarrassing moment? If not, why do I think others would change their opinion of me?

It is not possible to go through life without experiencing embarrassing moments. Decatastrophizing embarrassment will help you accept these inevitable moments as a fact of life. If you are more accepting of embarrassment, and see it as an uncomfortable but momentary state, you won't need to relitigate the past.

## 4. A Different Lens

We've seen that post-event processing can't give you any certainty about what you did or didn't do in the past. But a second problem is post-event processing's focus on the past rather than the present or future, which means it's not solution based. Because of these inherent flaws in post-event processing, it only increases anxiety.

Hana worked on developing a more practical, realistic alternative to her fear of offending others. Let's say she has a rather sharp exchange with a salesperson at her favorite clothing retailer. As she's driving home, she feels guilty about the interaction and starts ruminating on whether she offended the salesperson (post-event processing). She goes over and over the interaction trying to determine whether she was simply being assertive or was she rude and offensive. The more she ruminates on the interaction, the more her anxiety builds. She wonders if she should go back to the store and apologize to the salesperson. But somehow that seems strange, embarrassing, and fruitless. The salesperson deals with hundreds of people and will quickly forget about her. So rather than continue with her post-event processing, Hana decides to take a different approach. She will intentionally be more pleasant, positive, and complimentary to service people. This would turn the whole "rudeness incident" into a positive learning experience.

Often there is nothing you can do about a past remark or action that you regret. You can't take back a remark you now regret, and an apology is only helpful when you really did offend, hurt, or embarrass another person. Consider how you could respond differently to the following situations.

- **Embarrass yourself:** You make an inappropriate, inaccurate, or disrespectful remark and now you feel embarrassed. Rather than avoid people, you intentionally engage with them. If someone mentions your embarrassing remark, you state your regrets, acknowledge you made a mistake, and then return to the present, leaving "the past with the past." (It won't be your last mistake!)

- **Rude, offensive remark:** Again you continue to interact with the persons you may have offended. You treat them in a positive, respectful, and affirming manner. If the offense is mentioned, you express your regrets and offer an apology, but you then continue being inclusive of the person in your social interactions. You might even have to endure some slights from this individual but with time this will pass.

- **Criticism/disapproval of others:** You accept the criticism and consider whether there is anything you can learn from it. In this way, you are turning the criticism into a positive learning experience rather than a personal attack. Some criticism is so unjustified that nothing positive can be taken from it. If you can get some benefit from the criticism, you might thank the person for pointing out the shortcoming. For disapproval, you'll be yourself and continue to interact with the "disapproving people." If they continue to give off "disapproving vibes," you reduce your contact with them and spend more time with people who are affirming.

You'll notice that adopting a different lens means focusing on what can be done in the present rather than getting caught in fruitless rumination of the past. Being proactive, focused on the present can reduce anxiety. Getting caught in the endless cycle of post-event processing will only increase anxiety.

## What You Can Do

Hana's post-event processing was driven by a fear of offending others and causing them to feel shame. The fear that drives your post-event processing may be different. Maybe it's a fear of embarrassment, so your post-event rumination focuses on *did I say something embarrassing?* Or maybe you often feel embarrassed in situations and find you're focused on whether others shared in your embarrassment.

Or perhaps for you it's not embarrassment so much as a fear that you've made a poor or negative impression on others. Here the post-event rumination focuses on looking for evidence that you made a positive or negative impression on others. In this scenario you are probably falling into the error of mindreading; that is, trying to figure out what people really think about you.

Regardless of the fear that's fueling your post-event processing, you can use the exercises in this chapter to eliminate ruminating about the past. It'll take some diligent work and much patience but with practice, you can shift your focus from the past to the present. When you do this, you're taking an important step in reducing the negative effects of post-event processing on anxiety and worry.

# CONCLUSION

# This Is Your Anxiety

Congratulations! You've come to the end of our brief exposé of anxiety. Having gotten to this point, it's clear that you're looking for a fresh approach; some new ideas for dealing with unwanted fear, anxiety, or worry. Of course, anxiety is inevitable; it is an integral part of our emotional makeup. Because to be human is to feel anxious, anxiety is an emotion that can't be eliminated or entirely eradicated from our lives. Without anxiety, fear, and worry we'd be vulnerable to the many dangers, difficulties, and obstacles encountered in our daily lives. But like millions, you've come to realize your experience of anxiety has gotten out of hand. Compared to others, your experiences with anxiety are more frequent, intense, and debilitating, and it's now time to do something about it. It's time to take back your life and regain the happiness you once experienced.

*This Is What Anxiety Looks Like* was written with you in mind. It offered a solution-based perspective that started with explaining what it is that makes anxiety a debilitating problem for so many people. Each chapter focused on a different aspect of anxiety, one of the twelve basic psychological processes that cause the personal distress of feeling anxious. This was told to you through the lives of individuals I've treated in my practice—clinical composites that are intended to expose how anxiety interferes in our ability to live life to its fullest.

Everyone's experience of anxiety is somewhat different, but the underlying processes are similar. Anxiety, in its complexity, is like a puzzle. We all start with the same twelve pieces, but how we combine and arrange these pieces gives us a different experience of anxiety. Now that you've read through the book, I encourage you to review the chapters you read and figure out which of the twelve processes are most important to you. For some of you it may be anticipatory anxiety, catastrophizing, and avoidance that best define your experience. For others it might be fear of losing control, neutralization, and inflated responsibility. (If you experience panic attacks, look at the supplementary chapter online at http://www.newharbinger.com /53165. It offers interventions that focus on the physical symptoms of anxiety.)

Whatever the case, use what you've learned in *This Is What Anxiety Looks Like* to put together the pieces of your anxiety puzzle. Once you do this, you're ready to use the CBT exercises described in the previous chapters.

Each of the intervention strategies targets one of the core features of anxiety. You've been shown how the individuals featured in each chapter could use these interventions to overcome their problem with anxiety or worry. Now it's your turn. You can begin by developing your own intervention program from the descriptions provided in these chapters. You'll want to spend more time on the processes (pieces of your anxiety puzzle) that are most relevant for you. But you may also find that you need more detailed, step-by-step instruction on CBT to maximize its effectiveness. I've included a list of select resources at the end of this book that delve more deeply into the CBT approach to anxiety, fear, and worry.

For many of you this book represents a beginning. For others it may offer new hope in a struggle with anxiety you've been waging for years. Wherever you are on the path to better emotional health, it is my hope you've gained new insights and greater resolve to work on your CBT skills so you can reclaim what anxiety has taken from your life.

# Acknowledgments

Writing has always been one of the most solitary lines of work one can pursue. In the end what is written is always the purview of the author who wrote it. And yet, authorship is only part of the story. In reality, any publication is the result of teamwork, and this is especially true of *This Is What Anxiety Looks Like*.

I want to thank the staff and decision-makers at New Harbinger Publications for once again taking a chance on me and agreeing to provide their support, resources, and expertise in the publication of this book. I am especially grateful to Ryan Buresh, Acquisitions Editor at New Harbinger, who has been so kind and thoughtful throughout this project. This is now our fourth publication together, and each time his insights, support, and encouragement have been critical to the completion of a manuscript. Ryan is one of the most patient individuals I know, often gently working to convince me of the errors in my ways. I am also indebted to Vicraj Gill, Senior Editor at New Harbinger, for her methodical and perceptive editing of earlier drafts. She skillfully brought greater clarity, crispness, and understanding to many of the ideas I attempted to convey through these pages. I am also grateful to Amber Williams, copyeditor, and Sara Christian, cover designer, for their valuable contributions to this publication.

The knowledge and treatments conveyed in this book are the result of the work of many brilliant researchers, clinicians, and educators in the fields of clinical psychology and psychiatry. But of all the individuals who have been so influential throughout my career, one person stands out in particular. That is Dr. Aaron T. Beck, the pioneer of cognitive behavioral therapy

(CBT). It has been my honor and privilege to be mentored by Dr. Beck, and to coauthor several publications with him. Much of what you find in these pages is infused with his groundbreaking knowledge and treatment of anxiety. Also, it is my great fortune to have Bob Diforio as my literary agent. In this and other publications, he has given me a unique blend of support, encouragement, and wise counsel. Like with so many of my past writing projects, Bob played a key role in the current team effort and for this I am truly grateful. Lastly, I am indebted to Nancy Nason-Clark, my spouse of forty-six years, an academic and scholar in her own right, who continues to encourage and inspire.

# Additional Resources

Maybe *This Is What Anxiety Looks Like* is your first self-help on CBT for anxiety and worry. You've tried many of the exercises presented in these chapters, but you think you'd benefit from a more detailed, step-by-step instruction in the cognitive-behavioral approach to anxiety. Many people benefit from workbooks that have numerous worksheets designed to make CBT interventions more effective. If you are wondering what to read next, consider the following selected list of recommended resources, presented alphabetically by author.

Clark, D. A. 2018. *The Anxious Thoughts Workbook: Skills to Overcome the Unwanted Intrusive Thoughts That Drive Anxiety, Obsessions, and Depression.* Oakland, CA: New Harbinger Publications.

Clark, D. A., and A. T. Beck. 2023. *The Anxiety and Worry Workbook: The Cognitive Behavioral Solution,* 2nd ed. New York: Guilford Press.

Greenberger, D., and A. C. Padesky. 2015. *Mind Over Mood: Change How You Feel by Changing the Way You Think,* 2nd ed. New York: Guilford Press.

Hofmann, S. G. 2020. *The Anxiety Skills Workbook: Simple CBT and Mindfulness Strategies for Overcoming Anxiety, Fear, and Worry.* Oakland, CA: New Harbinger Publications.

Leahy, R. L. 2005. *The Worry Cure: Seven Steps to Stop Worry from Stopping You.* New York: Harmony Books.

Norton, P. J., and M. M. Antony. 2021. *The Anti-Anxiety Program,* 2nd ed. New York: Guilford Press.

Seif, M. N., and S. M. Winston. 2019. *Needing to Know for Sure: A CBT-Based Guide to Overcoming Compulsive Checking and Reassurance Seeking.* Oakland, CA: New Harbinger Publications.

Winston, S. M., and M. N. Seif. 2022. *Overcoming Anticipatory Anxiety: A CBT Guide for Moving Past Chronic Indecisiveness, Avoidance, and Catastrophic Thinking.* Oakland, CA: New Harbinger Publications.

**David A. Clark, PhD**, is a clinical psychologist, and professor emeritus at the University of New Brunswick in Canada. He is author of several books on depression and anxiety, including *Overcoming Obsessive Thoughts*, *The Anxiety and Worry Workbook*, *The Anxious Thoughts Workbook*, and *The Negative Thoughts Workbook*. He has coauthored several books with the pioneer of cognitive behavioral therapy (CBT), Aaron T. Beck, including *Cognitive Therapy for Anxiety Disorders*.

# Real change *is* possible

For more than fifty years, New Harbinger has published proven-effective self-help books and pioneering workbooks to help readers of all ages and backgrounds improve mental health and well-being, and achieve lasting personal growth. In addition, our spirituality books offer profound guidance for deepening awareness and cultivating healing, self-discovery, and fulfillment.

Founded by psychologist Matthew McKay and Patrick Fanning, New Harbinger is proud to be an independent, employee-owned company. Our books reflect our core values of integrity, innovation, commitment, sustainability, compassion, and trust. Written by leaders in the field and recommended by therapists worldwide, New Harbinger books are practical, accessible, and provide real tools for real change.

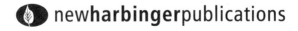 **newharbinger**publications

# MORE BOOKS from
# NEW HARBINGER PUBLICATIONS

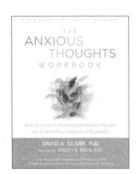
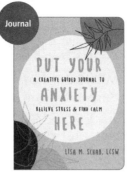
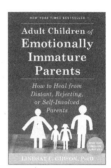
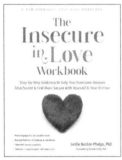
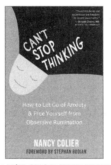
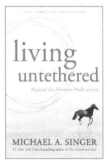

# Did you know there are **free tools** you can download for this book?

Free tools are things like **worksheets, guided meditation exercises**, and **more** that will help you get the most out of your book.

You can download free tools for this book—whether you bought or borrowed it, in any format, from any source—from the New Harbinger website. All you need is a NewHarbinger.com account. Just use the URL provided in this book to view the free tools that are available for it. Then, click on the "download" button for the free tool you want, and follow the prompts that appear to log in to your NewHarbinger.com account and download the material.

You can also save the free tools for this book to your **Free Tools Library** so you can access them again anytime, just by logging in to your account! Just look for this button on the book's free tools page.

**+ Save this to my free tools library**